Lippincott
Photo Atlas
of Medication
Administration

Lippincott
Photo Atlas
of Medication
Administration

···

Fifth Edition

Pamela Lynn, MSN, RN

Instructor
Gwynedd Mercy University
Frances M. Maguire School of Nursing and Health Professions
Gwynedd Valley, Pennsylvania

. Wolters Kluwer

Philadelphia · Baltimore · New York · London
Buenos Aires · Hong Kong · Sydney · Tokyo

Publisher: Lisa McAllister
Executive Editor: Sherry Dickinson
Product Developmental Editor: Christine Abshire
Editorial Assistant: Dan Reilly
Marketing Manager: Dean Karampelas
Production Project Manager: Joan Sinclair
Design Coordinator: Holly Reid McLaughlin
Illustration Coordinator: Jennifer Clements
Manufacturing Coordinator: Karin Duffield
Prepress Vendor: Aptara, Inc.

Fifth edition

9 8 7 6 5 4 3 2

Printed in China

ISBN: 9781451194319

LWW.com

Contents

Contents

SKILL 1 | ADMINISTERING ORAL MEDICATIONS

Drugs given orally are intended for absorption in the stomach and small intestine. The oral route is the most commonly used route of administration. It is usually the most convenient and comfortable route for the patient. After oral administration, drug action has a slower onset and a more prolonged, but less potent, effect than other routes.

DELEGATION CONSIDERATIONS

The administration of oral medications is not delegated to nursing assistive personnel (NAP) or to unlicensed assistive personnel (UAP) in the acute care setting. The administration of specified oral medications to stable patients in some long-term care settings may be delegated to nursing assistive personnel (NAP) or unlicensed assistive personnel (UAP) who have received appropriate training. Depending on the state's nurse practice act and the organization's policies and procedures, the administration of oral medications may be delegated to licensed practical/vocational nurses (LPN/LVNs). The decision to delegate must be based on careful analysis of the patient's needs and circumstances, as well as the qualifications of the person to whom the task is being delegated.

EQUIPMENT

- Medication in disposable cup or oral syringe
- Liquid (e.g., water, juice) with straw, if not contraindicated
- Medication cart or tray
- Computer-generated Medication Administration Record (CMAR) or Medication Administration Record (MAR)
- PPE, as indicated

ASSESSMENT

Assess the appropriateness of the drug for the patient. Review medical history, allergy, assessment, and laboratory data that may influence drug administration. Assess the patient's ability to swallow medications; check the gag reflex, if indicated. If the patient cannot swallow, is NPO, does not have gag reflex, or is experiencing nausea or vomiting, withhold the medication, notify the primary care provider, and complete proper documentation. Assess the patient's knowledge of the medication. If the patient has a knowledge deficit about the medication, this may be the appropriate time to begin education about the medication. If the medication may affect the patient's vital signs, assess them before administration. If the medication is for pain relief, assess the patient's pain level before and after administration. Verify the patient name, dose, route, and time of administration.

NURSING DIAGNOSIS

Determine related factors for the nursing diagnoses based on the patient's current status. Appropriate nursing diagnoses may include:

- Impaired Swallowing
- Deficient Knowledge
- Risk for Aspiration

OUTCOME IDENTIFICATION AND PLANNING

The expected outcome to achieve when administering an oral medication is that the patient will swallow the medication. Other outcomes that may be appropriate include the following: the patient will experience the desired effect from the medication; the patient will not aspirate; the patient experiences decreased anxiety; the patient does not experience adverse effects; and the patient understands and complies with the medication regimen.

IMPLEMENTATION

ACTION	RATIONALE
1. Gather equipment. Check each medication order against the original in the medical record, according to facility policy. Clarify any inconsistencies. Check the patient's medical record for allergies.	This comparison helps to identify errors that may have occurred when orders were transcribed. The primary care provider's order is the legal record of medication orders for each facility.
2. Know the actions, special nursing considerations, safe dose ranges, purpose of administration, and adverse effects of the medications to be administered. Consider the appropriateness of the medication for this patient.	This knowledge aids the nurse in evaluating the therapeutic effect of the medication in relation to the patient's disorder and can also be used to educate the patient about the medication.

(continued)

SKILL 1 ADMINISTERING ORAL MEDICATIONS continued

ACTION	RATIONALE
3. Perform hand hygiene.	Hand hygiene prevents the spread of microorganisms.
4. Move the medication cart to the outside of the patient's room or prepare for administration in the medication area.	Organization facilitates error-free administration and saves time.
5. Unlock the medication cart or drawer. Enter pass code into the computer and scan employee identification, if required.	Locking the cart or drawer safeguards each patient's medication supply. Hospital accrediting organizations require medication carts to be locked when not in use. Entering pass code and scanning ID allows only authorized users into the computer system and identifies the user for documentation by the computer.
6. **Prepare medications for one patient at a time.**	This prevents errors in medication administration.
7. Read the CMAR/MAR and select the proper medication from the unit stock or patient's medication drawer.	This is the *first* check of the medication label.
8. Compare the medication label with the CMAR/MAR (Figure 1). Check expiration dates and perform calculations, if necessary. Scan the bar code on the package, if required.	This is the *second* check of the label. Verify calculations with another nurse to ensure safety, if necessary.
9. Prepare the required medications:	
a. *Unit dose packages:* Place unit dose-packaged medications in a disposable cup. **Do not open the wrapper until at the bedside.** Keep opioids and medications that require special nursing assessments in a separate container.	Wrapper is kept intact because the label is needed for an additional safety check. Special assessments may be required before giving certain medications. These may include assessing vital signs and checking laboratory test results.
b. *Multidose containers:* When removing tablets or capsules from a multidose bottle, pour the necessary number into the bottle cap and then place the tablets or capsules in a medication cup. Break only scored tablets, if necessary, to obtain the proper dosage. Do not touch tablets or capsules with hands.	Pouring medication into the cap allows for easy return of excess medication to the bottle. Pouring tablets or capsules into your hand is unsanitary.
c. *Liquid medication in multidose bottle:* When pouring liquid medications out of a multidose bottle, hold the bottle so the label is against the palm. Use the appropriate measuring device when pouring liquids, and read the amount of medication at the bottom of the meniscus at eye level (Figure 2). Wipe the lip of the bottle with a paper towel.	Liquid that may drip onto the label makes the label difficult to read. Accuracy is possible when the appropriate measuring device is used and then read accurately.

FIGURE 1 Comparing medication label with CMAR.

FIGURE 2 Measuring at eye level. *(Photo by B. Proud.)*

ACTION	RATIONALE
10. Depending on facility policy, the third check of the label may occur at this point. If so, when all medications for one patient have been prepared, recheck the labels with the CMAR/MAR before taking the medications to the patient.	This *third* check ensures accuracy and helps to prevent errors. *Note:* Many facilities require the third check to occur at the bedside, after identifying the patient and before administration.
11. Replace any multidose containers in the patient's drawer or unit stock. **Lock the medication cart before leaving it.**	Locking the cart or drawer safeguards the patient's medication supply. Hospital accrediting organizations require medication carts to be locked when not in use.
12. Transport medications to the patient's bedside carefully, and keep the medications in sight at all times.	Careful handling and close observation prevent accidental or deliberate disarrangement of medications.
13. **Ensure that the patient receives the medications at the correct time.**	Check agency policy, which may allow for administration within a period of 30 minutes before or 30 minutes after the designated time.
14. Perform hand hygiene and put on PPE, if indicated.	Hand hygiene and PPE prevent the spread of microorganisms. PPE is required based on transmission precautions.
15. **Identify the patient. Compare the information with the CMAR/MAR. The patient should be identified using at least two methods** (The Joint Commission, 2013):	Identifying the patient ensures the right patient receives the medications and helps prevent errors. The patient's room number or physical location is not used as an identifier (The Joint Commission, 2013). Replace the identification band if it is missing or inaccurate in any way.
a. Check the name on the patient's identification band (Figure 3).	
b. Check the identification number on the patient's identification band.	
c. Check the birth date on the patient's identification band.	
d. Ask the patient to state his or her name and birth date, based on facility policy.	This requires a response from the patient, but illness and strange surroundings often cause patients to be confused.
16. **Complete necessary assessments before administering medications. Check the patient's allergy bracelet or ask the patient about allergies. Explain the purpose and action of each medication to the patient.**	Assessment is a prerequisite to administration of medications.
17. Scan the patient's bar code on the identification band, if required (Figure 4).	The bar code provides an additional check to ensure that the medication is given to the right patient.

FIGURE 3 Comparing patient's name and identification number with CMAR.

FIGURE 4 Scanning bar code on patient's identification bracelet. *(Photo by B. Proud.)*

(continued)

SKILL 1   ADMINISTERING ORAL MEDICATIONS   continued

ACTION	RATIONALE
18. Based on facility policy, the third check of the medication label may occur at this point. If so, recheck the label with the CMAR/MAR before administering the medications to the patient.	Many facilities require the *third* check to occur at the bedside, after identifying the patient and before administration. If facility policy directs the *third* check at this time, this *third* check ensures accuracy and helps prevent errors.
19. Assist the patient to an upright or lateral (side-lying) position.	Swallowing is facilitated by proper positioning. An upright or side-lying position protects the patient from aspiration.
20. Administer medications:	
a. Offer water or other permitted fluids with pills, capsules, tablets, and some liquid medications.	Liquids facilitate swallowing of solid drugs. Some liquid drugs are intended to adhere to the pharyngeal area, in which case liquid is not offered with the medication.
b. Ask whether the patient prefers to take the medications by hand or in a cup.	This encourages the patient's participation in taking the medications.
21. **Remain with the patient until each medication is swallowed. Never leave medication at the patient's bedside (Figure 5).**	Unless you have seen the patient swallow the drug, the drug cannot be recorded as administered. The patient's chart is a legal record. Medications can be left at the bedside only with a prescriber's order.

FIGURE 5 Remaining with patient until each medication is swallowed.

22. Assist the patient to a comfortable position. Remove PPE, if used. Perform hand hygiene.	Promotes patient comfort. Proper removal of PPE prevents transmission of microorganisms. Hand hygiene deters the spread of microorganisms.
23. Document the administration of the medication immediately after administration. See Documentation section below.	Timely documentation helps to ensure patient safety.
24. Evaluate the patient's response to the medication within the appropriate time frame.	The patient needs to be evaluated for therapeutic and adverse effects from the medication.

EVALUATION   The expected outcomes are met when the patient swallows the medication, does not aspirate, verbalizes an understanding of the medication, experiences the desired effect from the medication, and does not experience adverse effects.

DOCUMENTATION

Guidelines   Record each medication immediately after it is administered on the CMAR/MAR or record using the required format. Include the date and time of administration (Figure 6). If using a bar-code system, medication administration is automatically recorded when the bar code is scanned. PRN medications require documentation of the reason for administration. Prompt recording avoids the possibility of accidentally repeating the administration of the drug. If the drug was refused or omitted, record this in the appropriate area on the medication record and notify the primary care provider. This verifies the reason medication was omitted and ensures that the primary care provider is aware of the patient's condition. Recording administration of an opioid may require additional documentation on a controlled-substance record, stating drug count and other specific information. A record of fluid intake and output measurement is required.

FIGURE 6 Recording each medication administered on CMAR.

Sample Documentation

DocuCare **Practice documenting medication administration in** *Lippincott DocuCare.*

<u>8/6/15</u> 0835 Patient states he is having constant stabbing leg pains. Rates pain as an 8/10. Percocet 2 tabs administered.

—K. Sanders, RN

<u>8/6/15</u> 0905 Patient resting comfortably. Rates leg pain as a 1/10.

—K. Sanders, RN

<u>8/6/15</u> 1300 Patient states he does not want pain medication, despite return of leg pain. States, "It made me feel woozy last time." Feelings discussed with patient. Patient agrees to take Percocet 1 tab at this time.

—K. Sanders, RN

<u>8/6/15</u> 1320 Percocet, 1 tablet given PO.

—K. Sanders, RN

UNEXPECTED SITUATIONS AND ASSOCIATED INTERVENTIONS

- *Patient states that it feels like medication is lodged in throat:* Offer patient more fluids to drink. If allowed, offer the patient bread or crackers to help move the medication to the stomach.
- *It is unclear whether the patient swallowed the medication:* Check in the patient's mouth, under tongue, and between cheek and gum. Patients with altered mental status may not be aware that the medication was not swallowed. Also, patients may "cheek" medications to avoid taking the medication or to save it for later use. Watch patients requiring suicide precautions closely to ensure that they are not "cheeking" the medication or hiding it in the mouth. These patients may be trying to accumulate a large amount of medication to take all at once in a suicide attempt. Substance abusers may cheek medication to accumulate a large amount to take all at once so that they may feel a high from medication.
- *Patient vomits immediately or shortly after receiving oral medication:* Assess vomit, looking for pills or fragments. Do not re-administer medication without notifying primary care provider. If a whole pill is seen and can be identified, the primary care provider may ask that the medication be administered again. If a pill is not seen or medications cannot be identified, do not re-administer the medication in order to prevent the patient from receiving too large a dose.
- *Child refuses to take oral medications:* Some medications may be mixed in a small amount of food, such as pudding or ice cream. Do not add the medication to liquids because the medication may alter the taste of liquids; if child then refuses to drink the rest of the liquid, you will not know how much of the medication was ingested. Use creativity when devising ways to administer medications to a child. See the section below, Infant and Child Considerations, for suggestions.

(continued)

SKILL 1 ADMINISTERING ORAL MEDICATIONS continued

- *Capsule or tablet falls to the floor during administration:* Discard and obtain a new dose for administration. This prevents contamination and transmission of microorganisms.
- *Patient refuses medication:* Explore the reason for the patient's refusal. Review the rationale for using the drug and any other information that may be appropriate. If you are unable to administer the medication despite education and discussion, document the omission according to facility policy and notify the primary care provider.

SPECIAL CONSIDERATIONS

General Considerations

- Some liquid medication preparations, such as suspensions, require agitation to ensure even distribution of medication in the solution. Be familiar with the specific requirements for medications you are administering.
- Place medications intended for sublingual absorption under the patient's tongue. Instruct the patient to allow the medication to dissolve completely. Reinforce the importance of not swallowing the medication tablet.
- Some oral medications are provided in powdered forms. Verify the correct liquid in which to dissolve the medication for administration. This information is usually included on the package. Verify any unclear instructions with a pharmacist or medication reference. If there is more than one possible liquid in which to dissolve the medication, include the patient in the decision process; patients may find one choice more palatable than another.
- Ongoing assessment is an important part of nursing care for both evaluation of patient response to administered medications and early detection of adverse effects. If an adverse effect is suspected, withhold further medication doses and notify the patient's primary care provider. Additional intervention is based on type of reaction and patient assessment.
- If the patient questions a medication order or states the medication is different from the usual dose, always recheck and clarify with the original order and/or primary care provider before giving the medication.
- If the patient's level of consciousness is altered or his or her swallowing is impaired, check with the primary care provider to clarify the route of administration or alternative forms of medication. This may also be a solution for a pediatric or a confused patient who is refusing to take a medication.
- Patients with poor vision can request large-type labels on medication containers. A magnifying lens also may be helpful.
- Provide written medication information to reinforce discussion and education in the appropriate language, if the patient is literate. If the patient is unable to read, provide written information to family or significant other, if appropriate. Written information should be at a 5th-grade level to ensure ease of understanding.
- If the patient has difficulty swallowing tablets, it may be appropriate to crush the medication to facilitate administration. However, not all medications can be crushed or altered; long-acting and slow-release drugs are examples of medications that cannot be crushed. Therefore, it is important to consult a medication reference and/or pharmacist. If the medication can be crushed, use a pill-crusher or mortar and pestle to grind the tablet into a powder. Crush each pill one at a time. Dissolve the powder with water or other recommended liquid in a liquid medication cup, keeping each medication separate from the others. Keep the package label with the medication cup for future comparison of information. Combine the crushed medication with a small amount of soft food, such as applesauce or pudding, to facilitate administration.

Infant and Child Considerations

- Special devices, such as oral syringes and calibrated nipples, are available in a pharmacy to ensure accurate dose calculations for young children and infants.
- Some creative ways to administer medications to children include the following: have a "tea party" with medicine cups; place oral syringe (without needle) or dropper in the space between the cheek and gum and slowly administer the medication; save a special treat for after the medication administration (e.g., movie, playroom time, or a special food, if allowed).
- The Institute for Safe Medication Practices (ISMP) and the U.S. Food and Drug Administration (FDA) have received reports of infants choking on the plastic caps that fit on the end of syringes when used to administer oral medications. They recommend the following: Remove and dispose of caps before giving syringes to patients or families, caution family caregivers to dispose of caps on syringes they buy over the counter, and report any problems with syringe caps to the FDA. Companies manufacture syringes labeled "oral use" without the caps on them (ISMP, 2012b; FDA, 2012d).

Older Adult Considerations

- Older patients with arthritis may have difficulty opening childproof caps. On request, the pharmacist can substitute a cap that is easier to open. A rubber band twisted around the cap may provide a more secure grip for older patients.
- Consider large-print written medication information, when appropriate.
- Physiologic changes associated with the aging process, including decreased gastric motility, muscle mass, acid production, and blood flow, can affect patient's response to medication, including drug absorption and increased risk of adverse effects. Older adults are more likely to take multiple drugs, so drug interactions in the older adult are a very real and dangerous problem.

Home Care Considerations

- Encourage the patient to discard expired prescription medications based on label instructions or community guidelines.
- Discuss safe storage of medications when there are children and pets in the home environment.
- Discuss with parents the difference in over-the-counter medications made for infants and medications made for children. Many times parents do not realize that there are different strengths to the actual medications, leading to under- or overdosing.
- Encourage patients to carry a card listing all medications they take, including dosage and frequency, in case of an emergency.
- Discuss the importance of using an appropriate measuring device for liquid medications. Caution patients not to use eating utensils for measuring medications; use a liquid medication cup, oral syringe, or measuring spoon to provide accurate dosing.

EVIDENCE FOR PRACTICE ▶

MEDICATION ERRORS

Medication errors occur frequently and are a serious problem in health care. Medication errors may have serious consequences. Health care providers, including nurses, have a responsibility to prevent medication errors. What nursing practices may help improve the medication administration process?

Related Research

Murphy, M., & While, A. (2012). Medication administration practices among children's nurses: A survey. *British Journal of Nursing, 21*(15), 928–933.

This study investigated the medication administration practices of children's nurses to identify practices that may improve the medication administration process. Clinical staff working in all areas in a children's hospital were surveyed about medication errors and medication administration practices. Nurses identified interruptions in the medication process, a heavy workload, and fatigue as contributing factors to medication errors. In addition, the authors identified inadequate knowledge and skills and a failure to comply with hospital policy as additional contributing factors. The authors concluded that a lack of adherence to hospital policy and the frequency of interruptions in the medication administration process are important practices that require change.

Relevance to Nursing Practice

Medication administration is an important nursing responsibility. Nurses need to be aware of the factors that contribute to medication errors and work to reduce these factors in their practice. Nurses have a responsibility to be familiar with, and conform to, facility policies, as well as to maintain professional competency in regard to current and best practice guidelines. In addition, nurses should strive to work with facilities to ensure the provision of correct environment where interruptions and distractions can be kept to a minimum during all stages of the medication administration process.

(continued)

SKILL 1 ADMINISTERING ORAL MEDICATIONS continued

EVIDENCE FOR PRACTICE ▶

MEDICATION MANAGEMENT IN OLDER ADULTS

Older adults are often prescribed multiple medications. Low health literacy can affect the understanding of complex medication regimens by older adults. What nursing interventions can be used to address low health literacy and improve medication use among older adults?

Related Research

Martin, D., Kripalani, S., & DuRapau, J.J. (2012). Improving medication management among at-risk older adults. *Journal of Gerontological Nursing*, *38*(6), 24–34.

Community-dwelling older adults in this study were enrolled at an inner-city adult day center. Participants completed a baseline measure of health literacy, medication self-efficacy, and medication adherence. They were provided with a personalized, illustrated daily medication schedule. Six weeks later, their medication self-efficacy and adherence were assessed. Among the 20 participants in this pilot study, 70% had high likelihood of limited health literacy and took an average of 13.2 prescription medications. Both self-efficacy and medication adherence increased significantly after provision of the personalized illustrated daily medication schedule. All participants rated the schedules as very helpful in terms of helping them remember the medication's purpose and dosing. The authors concluded that illustrated daily medication schedules improve medication self-efficacy and adherence among at-risk community-dwelling older adults.

Relevance to Nursing Practice

Patient education is an important nursing responsibility. Nurses need to be creative and diligent in their approach to meeting the needs of their patients. Simple interventions, such as illustrated written schedules, along with explanation, can improve patient understanding and compliance.

SKILL 2 ADMINISTERING MEDICATIONS VIA A GASTRIC TUBE

Patients with a gastrointestinal tube (nasogastric, nasointestinal, percutaneous endoscopic gastrostomy [PEG], or jejunostomy [J] tube) often receive medication through the tube. Use liquid medications, when possible, because they are readily absorbed and less likely to cause tube occlusions. Certain solid dosage medications can be crushed and combined with liquid. Crush each pill, one at a time, to a fine powder and mix with 15 to 30 mL of water before delivery through the tube, keeping each medication separate from the others. Also, certain capsules may be opened, emptied into liquid, and administered through the tube (Toedter Williams, 2008). Not all medications can be crushed or altered; long-acting and slow-release drugs are examples of medications that cannot be crushed. Check manufacturer's recommendations and/or with a pharmacist to verify. Keep the package label with the medication cup for future comparison of information.

DELEGATION CONSIDERATIONS

The administration of medications via a gastric tube is not delegated to nursing assistive personnel (NAP) or to unlicensed assistive personnel (UAP). Depending on the state's nurse practice act and the organization's policies and procedures, the administration of medications via a gastric tube may be delegated to licensed practical/vocational nurses (LPN/LVNs). The decision to delegate must be based on careful analysis of the patient's needs and circumstances, as well as the qualifications of the person to whom the task is being delegated.

EQUIPMENT	• Irrigation set (60-mL syringe and irrigation container) • Medications • Water (gastrostomy tubes) or sterile water (naso-gastric [NG] tubes), according to facility policy	• Gloves • Additional PPE, as indicated

ASSESSMENT

Research each medication to be given, especially for mode of action, side effects, nursing implications, ability to be crushed, and whether the medication should be given with or without food. Verify patient name, dose, route, and time of administration. Also assess patient's knowledge of the medication and the reason for its administration. Auscultate the abdomen for evidence of bowel sounds. Palpate the abdomen for tenderness and distention. Ascertain the time of the patient's last bowel movement and measure abdominal girth, if appropriate.

NURSING DIAGNOSIS

Determine the related factors for the nursing diagnoses based on the patient's current status. Possible nursing diagnoses may include:

• Deficient Knowledge
• Risk for Injury

• Impaired Swallowing

OUTCOME IDENTIFICATION AND PLANNING

The expected outcome to achieve is that the patient receives the medication via the tube and experiences the intended effect of the medication. In addition, the patient verbalizes knowledge of the medications given; the patient remains free from adverse effects and injury; and the gastrointestinal tube remains patent.

IMPLEMENTATION

ACTION

RATIONALE

1. Gather equipment. Check each medication order against the original in the medical record, according to facility policy. Clarify any inconsistencies. Check the patient's chart for allergies.

This comparison helps to identify errors that may have occurred when orders were transcribed. The primary care provider's order is the legal record of medication orders for each facility.

2. Know the actions, special nursing considerations, safe dose ranges, purpose of administration, and adverse effects of the medications to be administered. Consider the appropriateness of the medication for this patient.

This knowledge aids the nurse in evaluating the therapeutic effect of the medication in relation to the patient's disorder and can also be used to educate the patient about the medication.

3. Perform hand hygiene.

Hand hygiene prevents the spread of microorganisms.

4. Move the medication cart to the outside of the patient's room or prepare for administration in the medication area.

Organization facilitates error-free administration and saves time.

5. Unlock the medication cart or drawer. Enter pass code into the computer and scan employee identification, if required.

Locking the cart or drawer safeguards each patient's medication supply. Hospital accrediting organizations require medication carts to be locked when not in use. Entering pass code and scanning ID allows only authorized users into the computer system and identifies the user for documentation by the computer.

6. Prepare medications for one patient at a time.

This prevents errors in medication administration.

7. Read the CMAR/MAR and select the proper medication from the unit stock or patient's medication drawer.

This is the *first* check of the label.

8. Compare the label with the CMAR/MAR. Check expiration dates and perform calculations, if necessary. Scan the bar code on the package, if required.

This is the *second* check of the label. Verify calculations with another nurse to ensure safety, if necessary.

(continued)

SKILL 2 ADMINISTERING MEDICATIONS VIA A GASTRIC TUBE   continued

ACTION	RATIONALE
9. Check to see if medications to be administered come in a liquid form. **If pills or capsules are to be given, check with pharmacy or drug reference to verify the ability to crush tablets or open capsules.**	To prevent the tube from becoming clogged, all medications should be given in liquid form whenever possible. Medications in extended-release formulations should not be crushed before administration.
10. Prepare medication.	Some medications require dissolution in liquid other than water. The label is needed for an additional safety check. Some medications require pre-administration assessments.
Pills: Using a pill crusher, crush each pill one at a time. Dissolve the powder with water or other recommended liquid in a liquid medication cup, keeping each medication separate from the others. Keep the package label with the medication cup, for future comparison of information.	
Liquid: When pouring liquid medications from a multidose bottle, hold the bottle with the label against the palm. Use the appropriate measuring device when pouring liquids, and read the amount of medication at the bottom of the meniscus at eye level. Wipe the lip of the bottle with a paper towel.	Liquid that may drip onto the label makes the label difficult to read. Accuracy is possible when the appropriate measuring device is used and then read accurately.
11. **Depending on facility policy, the third check of the label may occur at this point. If so, when all medications for one patient have been prepared, recheck the labels with the CMAR/MAR before taking the medications to the patient.**	This *third* check ensures accuracy and helps to prevent errors. *Note:* Many facilities require the *third* check to occur at the bedside, after identifying the patient and before administration.
12. Replace any multidose containers in the patient's drawer or unit stock.	Proper storage safeguards medications.
13. **Lock the medication cart before leaving it.**	Locking the cart or drawer safeguards the patient's medication supply. Hospital accrediting organizations require medication carts to be locked when not in use.
14. Transport medications to the patient's bedside carefully, and keep the medications in sight at all times.	Careful handling and close observation prevent accidental or deliberate disarrangement of medications.
15. **Ensure that the patient receives the medications at the correct time.**	Check agency policy, which may allow for administration within a period of 30 minutes before or 30 minutes after the designated time.
16. Perform hand hygiene and put on PPE, if indicated.	Hand hygiene and PPE prevent the spread of microorganisms. PPE is required based on transmission precautions.
17. **Identify the patient. Compare the information with the CMAR/MAR. The patient should be identified using at least two methods** (The Joint Commission, 2013):	Identifying the patient ensures the right patient receives the medications and helps prevent errors. The patient's room number or physical location is not used as an identifier (The Joint Commission, 2013). Replace the identification band if it is missing or inaccurate in any way.
a. Check the name on the patient's identification band.	
b. Check the identification number on the patient's identification band.	
c. Check the birth date on the patient's identification band.	
d. Ask the patient to state his or her name and birth date, based on facility policy.	This requires a response from the patient, but illness and strange surroundings often cause patients to be confused.
18. **Complete necessary assessments before administering medications. Check the patient's allergy bracelet or ask the patient about allergies. Explain what you are going to do, and the reason for doing it, to the patient.**	Assessment is a prerequisite to administration of medications. Explanation relieves anxiety and facilitates cooperation.

ACTION	RATIONALE

19. Scan the patient's bar code on the identification band, if required (Figure 1).

This provides an additional check to ensure that the medication is given to the right patient.

20. **Based on facility policy, the third check of the label may occur at this point. If so, recheck the labels with the CMAR/MAR before administering the medications to the patient.**

Many facilities require the *third* check to occur at the bedside, after identifying the patient and before administration. If facility policy directs the *third* check at this time, this *third* check ensures accuracy and helps to prevent errors.

21. Assist the patient to the high Fowler's position, unless contraindicated.

This reduces the risk of aspiration.

22. Put on gloves.

Gloves prevent contact with mucous membranes and body fluids.

23. If patient is receiving continuous tube feedings, pause the tube-feeding pump (Figure 2).

If the pump is not stopped, tube feeding will flow out of the tube and onto the patient.

FIGURE 1 Scanning bar code on the patient's identification bracelet. *(Photo by B. Proud.)*

FIGURE 2 Pausing feeding pump. *(Photo by B. Proud.)*

24. Pour the water into the irrigation container. Measure 30 mL of water. Apply clamp on feeding tube, if present. Alternately, pinch gastric tube below port with fingers, or position stopcock to correct direction. Open port on gastric tube delegated to medication administration (Figure 3) or disconnect tubing for feeding from gastric tube and place cap on end of feeding tubing.

Fluid is ready for flushing of the tube. Applying clamp, folding the tube over, and clamping, or the correct positioning of the stopcock prevents any backflow of gastric drainage. Covering end of feeding tubing prevents contamination.

25. **Check tube placement, depending on type of tube and facility policy.**

Tube placement must be confirmed before administering anything through the tube to avoid inadvertent instillation in the respiratory tract.

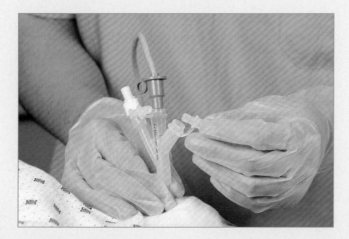

FIGURE 3 Pinching gastric tubing to prevent backflow of gastric drainage and opening medication administration port. *(Photo by B. Proud.)*

(*continued*)

SKILL 2 ADMINISTERING MEDICATIONS VIA A GASTRIC TUBE continued

ACTION

RATIONALE

26. Note the amount of any residual. Replace residual back into stomach, based on facility policy.

Research findings are inconclusive on the benefit of returning gastric volumes to the stomach or intestine to avoid fluid or electrolyte imbalance, which has been accepted practice. Consult agency policy concerning this practice (Bourgault, et al., 2007; Keithley & Swanson, 2004; Metheny, 2008).

27. Apply clamp on feeding tube, if present. Alternately, pinch the gastric tube below port with fingers, or position stop-cock to correct direction. Remove 60-mL syringe from gastric tube. Remove the plunger of the syringe. Reinsert the syringe in the gastric tube without the plunger. Pour 30 mL of water into the syringe (Figure 4). **Unclamp the tube and allow the water to enter the stomach via gravity infusion.**

Clamping prevents backflow of gastric drainage. Flushing the tube ensures that all the residual is cleared from the tube.

28. Administer the first dose of medication by pouring it into the syringe (Figure 5). Follow with a 5- to 10-mL water flush between medication doses. Follow the last dose of medication with 30 to 60 mL of water flush.

Flushing between medications prevents any possible interactions between the medications. Flushing at the end maintains tube patency, prevents blockage by medication particles, and ensures all doses enter the stomach.

FIGURE 4 Pouring water into syringe inserted in gastric tube. *(Photo by B. Proud.)*

FIGURE 5 Pouring medication into syringe inserted in gastric tube. *(Photo by B. Proud.)*

29. Clamp the tube, remove the syringe, and replace the feeding tubing. If a stopcock is used, position it to correct direction. If a tube medication port was used, cap the port. Unclamp the gastric tube and restart tube feeding, if appropriate for medications administered.

Some medications require the holding of the tube feeding for a certain period of time after administration. Consult a drug reference or a pharmacist.

30. Remove gloves. Assist the patient to a comfortable position. If receiving a tube feeding, the head of the bed must remain elevated at least 30 degrees.

Ensures patient comfort. Keeping the head of the bed elevated helps prevent aspiration.

31. Remove additional PPE, if used. Perform hand hygiene.

Removing PPE properly reduces the risk for infection transmission and contamination of other items. Hand hygiene prevents the spread of microorganisms.

32. Document the administration of the medication immediately after administration. See Documentation section below.

Timely documentation helps to ensure patient safety.

33. Evaluate the patient's response to the medication within the appropriate time frame.

The patient needs to be evaluated for therapeutic and adverse effects from the medication.

EVALUATION

The expected outcome is met when the patient receives the prescribed medications and experiences the intended effects of the medications administered. In addition, the patient demonstrates a patent and functioning gastric tube, verbalizes knowledge of the medications given, and remains free from adverse effects and injury.

DOCUMENTATION
Guidelines

Document the administration of the medication immediately after administration, including date, time, dose, and route of administration on the CMAR/MAR or record using the required format. If using a bar-code system, medication administration is automatically recorded when the bar code is scanned. PRN medications require documentation of the reason for administration. Prompt recording avoids the possibility of accidentally repeating the administration of the drug. Record the amount of gastric residual, if appropriate. Record the amount of liquid given on the intake and output record. If the drug was refused or omitted, record this in the appropriate area on the medication record and notify the primary care provider. This verifies the reason medication was omitted and ensures that the primary care provider is aware of the patient's condition.

UNEXPECTED SITUATIONS AND ASSOCIATED INTERVENTIONS

• *Medication enters tube and then tube becomes clogged:* Attach a 10-mL syringe onto end of tube. Pull back and then lightly apply pressure to plunger in a repetitive motion. This may dislodge the medication. If the medication does not move through the tube, notify the primary care provider. The tube may have to be replaced.

SPECIAL CONSIDERATIONS

• If medications are being administered via an NG tube that is attached to suction, the tube should remain clamped, off suction, for a period of time after medication administration. This allows for medication absorption before returning to suction. Check facility policy and drug reference for specific drug requirements.
• If necessary to use plunger in irrigation syringe to administer medications, instill gently and slowly. Gravity administration is considered best to avoid excess pressure.
• Give medications separately and flush with water between each drug. Some medications may interact with each other or become less effective if mixed with other drugs.
• If the patient is receiving tube feedings, review information about the drugs to be administered. Absorption of some drugs, such as phenytoin (Dilantin), is affected by tube feeding formulas. Discontinue a continuous tube feeding and leave the tube clamped for the required period of time before and after the medication has been given, according to the reference and facility protocol.
• Ongoing assessment is an important part of nursing care for both evaluation of patient response to administered medications and early detection of adverse effects. If an adverse effect is suspected, withhold further medication doses and notify the patient's primary care provider. Additional intervention is based on type of reaction and patient assessment.

SKILL 3   REMOVING MEDICATION FROM AN AMPULE

An **ampule** is a glass flask that contains a single dose of medication for parenteral administration. Because there is no way to prevent contamination of any unused portion of medication after the ampule is opened, discard any remaining medication if not all the medication is used for the prescribed dose. You must break the thin neck of the ampule to remove the medication.

DELEGATION CONSIDERATIONS

The preparation of medication from an ampule is not delegated to nursing assistive personnel (NAP) or to unlicensed assistive personnel (UAP). Depending on the state's nurse practice act and the organization's policies and procedures, the preparation of medication from an ampule may be delegated to a licensed practical/vocational nurse (LPN/LVN). The decision to delegate must be based on careful analysis of the patient's needs and circumstances, as well as the qualifications of the person to whom the task is being delegated.

(continued)

SKILL 3 REMOVING MEDICATION FROM AN AMPULE continued

EQUIPMENT	• Sterile syringe and filter needle • Ampule of medication • Small gauze pad • Computer-generated Medication Administration Record (CMAR) or Medication Administration Record (MAR)
ASSESSMENT	Assess the medication in the ampule for any particles or discoloration. Assess the ampule for any cracks or chips. Check expiration date before administering the medication. Verify patient name, dose, route, and time of administration. Assess the appropriateness of the drug for the patient. Review assessment and laboratory data that may influence drug administration.
NURSING DIAGNOSIS	Determine related factors for the nursing diagnoses based on the patient's current status. Appropriate nursing diagnoses may include: • Risk for Infection • Risk for Injury • Deficient Knowledge
OUTCOME IDENTIFICATION AND PLANNING	The expected outcome to achieve when removing medication from an ampule is that the medication will be removed in a sterile manner; it will be free from glass shards and the proper dose prepared.

IMPLEMENTATION

ACTION	RATIONALE
1. Gather equipment. Check the medication order against the original order in the medical record, according to facility policy. Clarify any inconsistencies. Check the patient's chart for allergies.	This comparison helps to identify errors that may have occurred when orders were transcribed. The primary care provider's order is the legal record of medication orders for each facility.
2. Know the actions, special nursing considerations, safe dose ranges, purpose of administration, and adverse effects of the medications to be administered. Consider the appropriateness of the medication for this patient.	This knowledge aids the nurse in evaluating the therapeutic effect of the medication in relation to the patient's disorder and can also be used to educate the patient about the medication.
3. Perform hand hygiene.	Hand hygiene prevents the spread of microorganisms.
4. Move the medication cart to the outside of the patient's room or prepare for administration in the medication area.	Organization facilitates error-free administration and saves time.
5. Unlock the medication cart or drawer. Enter pass code and scan employee identification, if required.	Locking the cart or drawer safeguards each patient's medication supply. Hospital accrediting organizations require medication carts to be locked when not in use. Entering pass code and scanning ID allows only authorized users into the computer system and identifies the user for documentation by the computer.
6. Prepare medications for one patient at a time.	This prevents errors in medication administration.
7. Read the CMAR/MAR and select the proper medication from unit stock or the patient's medication drawer.	This is the *first* check of the label.
8. Compare the label with the CMAR/MAR. Check expiration dates and perform calculations, if necessary. Scan the bar code on the package, if required.	This is the *second* check of the label. Verify calculations with another nurse to ensure safety, if necessary.

ACTION	RATIONALE

9. Tap the stem of the ampule (Figure 1) or twist your wrist quickly (Figure 2) while holding the ampule vertically.

This facilitates movement of medication in the stem to the body of the ampule.

10. Wrap a small gauze pad around the neck of the ampule.

This will protect your fingers from the glass as the ampule is broken.

FIGURE 1 Tapping stem of the ampule.

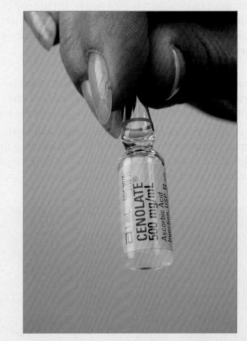

FIGURE 2 Twisting wrist quickly while holding ampule vertically.

11. Use a snapping motion to break off the top of the ampule along the scored line at its neck (Figure 3). **Always break away from your body.**

This protects your face and fingers from any shattered glass fragments.

FIGURE 3 Using a snapping motion to break top of ampule.

(continued)

SKILL 3 REMOVING MEDICATION FROM AN AMPULE continued

ACTION	RATIONALE

ACTION

12. Attach filter needle to syringe. Remove the cap from the filter needle by pulling it straight off.

13. Withdraw medication in the amount ordered plus a small amount more (approximately 30% more). **Do not inject air into the solution. While inserting the filter needle into the ampule, be careful not to touch the rim.** Use either of the following methods to withdraw the medication:

   a. Insert the tip of the needle into the ampule, which is upright on a flat surface, and withdraw fluid into the syringe (Figure 4). **Touch the plunger only at the knob.**

   b. Insert the tip of the needle into the ampule and invert the ampule. Keep the needle centered and not touching the sides of the ampule. Withdraw fluid into syringe (Figure 5). **Touch the plunger only at the knob.**

RATIONALE

Use of a filter needle prevents the accidental withdrawing of small glass particles with the medication. Pulling the cap off in a straight manner prevents accidental needlestick.

By withdrawing an additional small amount of medication, any air bubbles in the syringe can be displaced once the syringe is removed while allowing ample medication to remain in the syringe. The contents of the ampule are not under pressure; therefore, air is unnecessary and will cause the contents to overflow. The rim of the ampule is considered contaminated.

Handling the plunger only at the knob will keep the shaft of the plunger sterile.

Surface tension holds the fluids in the ampule when inverted. If the needle touches the sides or is removed and then reinserted into the ampule, surface tension is broken, and fluid runs out. Handling the plunger only at the knob will keep the shaft of the plunger sterile.

FIGURE 4 Withdrawing medication from upright ampule. *(Photo by B. Proud.)*

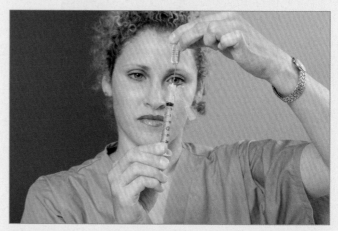

FIGURE 5 Withdrawing medication from inverted ampule. *(Photo by B. Proud.)*

14. Wait until the needle has been withdrawn to tap the syringe and expel the air carefully by pushing on the plunger. **Check the amount of medication in the syringe with the medication dose and discard any surplus, according to facility policy.**

15. **Depending on facility policy, the third check of the label may occur at this point. If so, when all medications for one patient have been prepared, recheck the labels with the CMAR/MAR before taking the medications to the patient.**

16. **Engage safety guard on filter needle and remove the needle. Discard the filter needle in a suitable container. Attach appropriate administration device to syringe.**

17. Discard the ampule in a suitable container.

18. Lock the medication cart before leaving it.

Ejecting air into the solution increases pressure in the ampule and can force the medication to spill out over the ampule. Ampules may have overfill. Careful measurement ensures that the correct dose is withdrawn.

This *third* check ensures accuracy and helps to prevent errors. *Note:* Many facilities require the *third* check to occur at the bedside, after identifying the patient and before administration.

The filter needle used to draw up medication should not be used to administer the medication. This will prevent any glass shards from entering the patient during administration.

Any medication that has not been removed from the ampule must be discarded because sterility of contents cannot be maintained in an opened ampule.

Locking the cart or drawer safeguards the patient's medication supply. Hospital accrediting organizations require medication carts to be locked when not in use.

ACTION	**RATIONALE**

19. Perform hand hygiene.

Hand hygiene deters the spread of microorganisms.

20. Proceed with administration, based on prescribed route.

See appropriate skill for prescribed route.

EVALUATION

The expected outcome is met when the medication is removed from the ampule in a sterile manner, is free from glass shards, and the proper dose is prepared.

DOCUMENTATION

Guidelines

It is not necessary to record the removal of the medication from the ampule. Prompt recording of administration of the medication is required immediately after it is administered.

UNEXPECTED SITUATIONS AND ASSOCIATED INTERVENTIONS

- *You cut yourself while trying to open the ampule:* Discard ampule in case contamination has occurred. Clean and bandage the wound and obtain a new ampule. Report according to facility policy.
- *All of medication was not removed from the stem and insufficient medication remains in body of ampule:* Discard ampule and drawn medication. Obtain a new ampule and start over. Medication in original ampule stem is considered contaminated once neck of ampule has been placed on a nonsterile surface.
- *You inject air into inverted ampule, spraying medication:* Wash hands to remove any medication. If any medication has gotten into eyes, perform eye irrigation. Obtain a new ampule for medication dose. Report injury, if appropriate, according to facility policy.
- *Medication is drawn up without using a filter needle:* Replace needle with a filter needle. Inject the medication through the filter needle into a new syringe and then administer to patient.
- *Plunger becomes contaminated before inserted into ampule:* Discard needle and syringe and start over. If plunger is contaminated after medication is drawn into the syringe, it is not necessary to discard and start over. The contaminated plunger will enter the barrel of the syringe when pushing the medication out and will not contaminate the medication.

SKILL 4 | REMOVING MEDICATION FROM A VIAL

A vial is a glass bottle with a self-sealing stopper through which medication is removed. For safety in transporting and storing, the vial top is usually covered with a soft metal cap that can be removed easily. The self-sealing stopper that is then exposed is the means of entrance into the vial. Single-dose vials are used once, and then discarded, regardless of the amount of the drug that is used from the vial. Multi-dose vials contain several doses of medication and can be used multiple times. The Centers for Disease Control and Prevention (CDC) recommends that medications packaged as multiuse vials be assigned to a single patient whenever possible (CDC, 2011). In addition, it is recommended that the top of the vial be cleaned before each entry, and that a new sterile needle and syringe are used for each entry. The medication contained in a vial can be in liquid or powder form. Powdered forms must be dissolved in an appropriate diluent before administration. The following skill reviews removing liquid medication from a vial. Refer to the accompanying Skill Variation for steps to reconstitute powdered medication.

DELEGATION CONSIDERATIONS

The preparation of medication from a vial is not delegated to nursing assistive personnel (NAP) or to unlicensed assistive personnel (UAP). Depending on the state's nurse practice act and the organization's policies and procedures, the preparation of medication from a vial may be delegated to licensed practical/vocational nurses (LPN/LVNs). The decision to delegate must be based on careful analysis of the patient's needs and circumstances, as well as the qualifications of the person to whom the task is being delegated.

(continued)

SKILL 4 REMOVING MEDICATION FROM A VIAL continued

EQUIPMENT

- Sterile syringe and needle or blunt cannula (size depends on medication being administered)
- Vial of medication
- Antimicrobial swab

- Second needle (optional)
- Filter needle (optional)
- Computer-generated Medication Administration Record (CMAR) or Medication Administration Record (MAR)

ASSESSMENT

Assess the medication in the vial for any discoloration or particles. Check expiration date before administering medication. Verify patient name, dose, route, and time of administration. Assess the appropriateness of the drug for the patient. Review assessment and laboratory data that may influence drug administration.

NURSING DIAGNOSIS

Determine related factors for the nursing diagnoses based on the patient's current status. Appropriate nursing diagnoses include:

- Risk for Infection
- Deficient Knowledge

- Risk for Injury

OUTCOME IDENTIFICATION AND PLANNING

The expected outcome to achieve when removing medication from a vial is withdrawal of the medication into a syringe in a sterile manner and preparation of the proper dose.

IMPLEMENTATION

ACTION	RATIONALE
1. Gather equipment. Check the medication order against the original order in the medical record, according to facility policy. Clarify any inconsistencies. Check the patient's chart for allergies.	This comparison helps to identify errors that may have occurred when orders were transcribed. The primary care provider's order is the legal record of medication orders for each facility.
2. Know the actions, special nursing considerations, safe dose ranges, purpose of administration, and adverse effects of the medications to be administered. Consider the appropriateness of the medication for this patient.	This knowledge aids the nurse in evaluating the therapeutic effect of the medication in relation to the patient's disorder and can also be used to educate the patient about the medication.
3. Perform hand hygiene.	Hand hygiene deters the spread of microorganisms.
4. Move the medication cart to the outside of the patient's room or prepare for administration in the medication area.	Organization facilitates error-free administration and saves time.
5. Unlock the medication cart or drawer. Enter pass code and scan employee identification, if required.	Locking the cart or drawer safeguards each patient's medication supply. Hospital accrediting organizations require medication carts to be locked when not in use. Entering pass code and scanning ID allows only authorized users into the system and identifies the user for documentation by the computer.
6. **Prepare medications for one patient at a time.**	This prevents errors in medication administration.
7. Read the CMAR/MAR and select the proper medication from unit stock or the patient's medication drawer.	This is the *first* check of the label.
8. Compare the label with the CMAR/MAR. Check expiration dates and perform calculations, if necessary. Scan the bar code on the package, if required.	This is the *second* check of the label. Verify calculations with another nurse to ensure safety, if necessary.
9. Remove the metal or plastic cap on the vial that protects the rubber stopper.	Cap needs to be removed to access medication in the vial.

ACTION

10. **Swab the rubber top with the antimicrobial swab and allow to dry.**

11. Remove the cap from the needle or blunt cannula by pulling it straight off. Touch the plunger only at the knob. Draw back an amount of air into the syringe that is equal to the specific dose of medication to be withdrawn. Some facilities require use of a filter needle when withdrawing premixed medication from multidose vials.

12. Hold the vial on a flat surface. Pierce the rubber stopper in the center with the needle tip and inject the measured air into the space above the solution (Figure 1). Do not inject air into the solution.

13. Invert the vial. **Keep the tip of the needle or blunt cannula below the fluid level (Figure 2).**

14. Hold the vial in one hand and use the other to withdraw the medication. **Touch the plunger only at the knob. Draw up the prescribed amount of medication while holding the syringe vertically and at eye level (Figure 3).**

RATIONALE

Antimicrobial swab removes surface bacterial contamination. Allowing the alcohol to dry prevents it from entering the vial on the needle.

Pulling the cap off in a straight manner prevents accidental needlestick injury. Handling the plunger only at the knob will keep the shaft of the plunger sterile. Because a vial is a sealed container, injection of an equal amount of air (before fluid is removed) is required to prevent the formation of a partial vacuum. If not enough air is injected, the negative pressure makes it difficult to withdraw the medication. Using a filter needle prevents any solid material from being withdrawn through the needle.

Air bubbled through the solution could result in withdrawal of an inaccurate amount of medication.

This prevents air from being aspirated into the syringe.

Handling the plunger only at the knob will keep the shaft of the plunger sterile. Holding the syringe at eye level facilitates accurate reading, and the vertical position makes removal of air bubbles from the syringe easy.

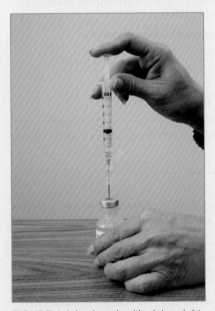

FIGURE 1 Injecting air with vial upright.

FIGURE 2 Positioning needle tip in solution.

FIGURE 3 Withdrawing medication at eye level.

15. If any air bubbles accumulate in the syringe, tap the barrel of the syringe sharply and move the needle past the fluid into the air space to re-inject the air bubble into the vial. Return the needle tip to the solution and continue withdrawal of the medication.

Removal of air bubbles is necessary to ensure an accurate dose of medication.

(continued)

SKILL 4 | REMOVING MEDICATION FROM A VIAL continued

ACTION	RATIONALE
16. After the correct dose is withdrawn, remove the needle from the vial and carefully replace the cap over the needle. **If a filter needle has been used to draw up the medication, remove it and attach the appropriate administration device.** Some facilities require changing the needle, if one was used to withdraw the medication, before administering the medication.	This prevents contamination of the needle and protects against accidental needlesticks. A one-handed recap method may be used as long as care is taken not to contaminate the needle during the process. A filter needle used to draw up medication should not be used to administer the medication to prevent any solid material from entering the patient. Changing the needle may be necessary because passing the needle through the stopper on the vial may dull the needle. In addition, it ensures the tip of the needle is free from medication residue, significantly reducing pain intensity associated with the injection (Ağaç & Güneş, 2010).
17. **Check the amount of medication in the syringe with the medication dose and discard any surplus.**	Careful measurement ensures that the correct dose is withdrawn.
18. **Depending on facility policy, the third check of the label may occur at this point. If so, when all medications for one patient have been prepared, recheck the labels with the CMAR/MAR before taking the medications to the patient.**	This *third* check ensures accuracy and helps to prevent errors. *Note:* Many facilities require the *third* check to occur at the bedside, after identifying the patient and before administration.
19. **If a multidose vial is being used, label the vial with the date and time opened, and store the vial containing the remaining medication according to facility policy.**	Because the vial is sealed, the medication inside remains sterile and can be used for future injections. Labeling the opened vials with a date and time limits its use after a specific time period.
20. Lock the medication cart before leaving it.	Locking the cart or drawer safeguards the patient's medication supply. Hospital accrediting organizations require medication carts to be locked when not in use.
21. Perform hand hygiene.	Hand hygiene deters the spread of microorganisms.
22. Proceed with administration, based on prescribed route.	See appropriate skill for prescribed route.

EVALUATION

The expected outcome is met when the medication is withdrawn into the syringe in a sterile manner and the proper dose is prepared.

DOCUMENTATION
Guidelines

It is not necessary to record the removal of the medication from the ampule. Prompt recording of administration of the medication is required immediately after it is administered.

UNEXPECTED SITUATIONS AND ASSOCIATED INTERVENTIONS

- *A piece of rubber stopper is noticed floating in the medication in the syringe:* Discard the syringe, needle, and vial. Obtain a new vial, syringe, and needle and prepare dose as ordered.
- *As needle attached to syringe filled with air is inserted into vial, the plunger is immediately pulled down:* If possible to withdraw medication, continue steps as explained above. If such a vacuum has formed that this is impossible, remove syringe and inject more air into the vial. This is caused by previous withdrawal of medication without the addition of air into the vial.
- *Plunger is contaminated before injecting air into vial:* Discard needle and syringe and start over.
- *Plunger is contaminated after medication is drawn into syringe:* It is not necessary to discard needle and syringe and start over. The contaminated plunger will enter the barrel of the syringe when pushing the medication out and will not contaminate the medication.

SKILL VARIATION   Reconstituting Powdered Medication in a Vial

Drugs that are unstable in liquid form are often provided in a dry powder form. The powder must be mixed with the correct amount of appropriate solution to prepare the medication for administration. Verify the correct amount and correct solution type for the specific medication prescribed. This information is found on the vial label, package insert, in a drug reference, an on-line pharmacy source, or from the pharmacist. To reconstitute powdered medication:

1. Gather equipment. Check the medication order against the original order in the medical record, according to agency policy.
2. Know the actions, special nursing considerations, safe dose ranges, purpose of administration, and adverse effects of the medications to be administered. Consider the appropriateness of the medication for this patient.

3. Perform hand hygiene.

4. Move the medication cart to the outside of the patient's room or prepare for administration in the medication area.
5. Unlock the medication cart or drawer. Enter pass code and scan employee identification, if required.
6. **Prepare medications for one patient at a time.**
7. Read the CMAR/MAR and select the proper medication and diluent from unit stock or from the patient's medication drawer. This is the *first* check of the medication label.
8. Compare the labels with the CMAR/MAR. This is the *second* check of the medication label. Check expiration dates and perform calculations, check medication calculation with another nurse. Scan the bar code on the package, if required.
9. Remove the metal or plastic cap on the medication vial and diluent vial that protects the self-sealing stoppers.

10. Swab the self-sealing tops with the antimicrobial swab and allow to dry.
11. **Draw up the appropriate amount of diluent into the syringe.**
12. Insert the needle or blunt cannula through the center of the self-sealing stopper on the powdered medication vial.
13. Inject the diluent into the powdered medication vial.
14. Remove the needle or blunt cannula from the vial and replace cap.
15. **Gently agitate the vial to mix the powdered medication and the diluent completely. Do not shake the vial.**
16. **Draw up the prescribed amount of medication while holding the syringe vertically and at eye level.**
17. After the correct dose is withdrawn, remove the needle from the vial and carefully replace the cap over the needle. **If a filter needle has been used to draw up the medication, remove it and attach the appropriate administration device.** Some facilities require changing the needle, if one was used to withdraw the medication, before administering the medication.
18. **Check the amount of medication in the syringe with the medication dose and discard any surplus.**
19. **Depending on facility policy, the third check of the label may occur at this point. If so, recheck the label with the CMAR/MAR before taking the medications to the patient.**
20. Lock the medication cart before leaving it.

21. Perform hand hygiene.

22. Proceed with administration, based on prescribed route.

SKILL 5   MIXING MEDICATIONS FROM TWO VIALS IN ONE SYRINGE

Preparation of medications in one syringe depends on how the medication is supplied. When using a single-dose vial and a multidose vial, air is injected into both vials and the medication in the multidose vial is drawn into the syringe first. This prevents the contents of the multidose vial from being contaminated with the medication in the single-dose vial. The CDC recommends that medications packaged as multiuse vials be assigned to a single patient whenever possible (CDC, 2011). In addition, it is recommended that the top of the vial be cleaned before each entry, and that a new sterile needle and syringe are used before each entry.

When considering mixing two medications in one syringe, you must ensure that the two drugs are compatible. Be aware of drug incompatibilities when preparing medications in one syringe. Certain medications, such as diazepam (Valium), are incompatible with other drugs in the same syringe. Incompatible drugs may become cloudy or form a precipitate in the syringe. Such medications are discarded and prepared again in separate syringes. Other drugs have limited compatibility and should be administered within 15 minutes of preparation. Mixing more than two drugs in one

(continued)

SKILL 5

MIXING MEDICATIONS FROM TWO VIALS IN ONE SYRINGE   continued

syringe is not recommended. If it must be done, contact the pharmacist to determine the compatibility of the three drugs, as well as the compatibility of their pH values and the preservatives that may be present in each drug. A drug-compatibility table should be available to nurses who are preparing medications.

Insulin, with many types available for use, is an example of a medication that may be combined together in one syringe for injection. Insulins vary in their onset and duration of action and are classified as rapid acting, short acting, intermediate acting, and long acting. Before administering any insulin, be aware of the onset time, peak, and duration of effects, and ensure that proper food is available. Be aware that some insulins, such as Lantus and Levemir, cannot be mixed with other insulins. Refer to a drug reference for a listing of the different types of insulin and action specific to each type. Insulin dosages are calculated in units. The scale commonly used is U100, which is based on 100 units of insulin contained in 1 mL of solution.

DELEGATION CONSIDERATIONS	The preparation of medication from two vials is not delegated to nursing assistive personnel (NAP) or to unlicensed assistive personnel (UAP). Depending on the state's nurse practice act and the organization's policies and procedures, the preparation of medication from two vials may be delegated to licensed practical/vocational nurses (LPN/LVNs). The decision to delegate must be based on careful analysis of the patient's needs and circumstances, as well as the qualifications of the person to whom the task is being delegated.
EQUIPMENT	The preparation of two types of insulin in one syringe is used as the example in the following procedure. • Two vials of medication (insulin in this example) • Sterile syringe (insulin syringe in this example) • Antimicrobial swabs • Computer-generated Medication Administration Record (CMAR) or Medication Administration Record (MAR)
ASSESSMENT	Determine the compatibility of the two medications. Not all insulin can be mixed together. For example, Lantus and Levemir cannot be mixed with another insulin. Assess the contents of each vial of insulin. It is very important to be familiar with the particular drug's properties to be able to assess the quality of the medication in the vial before withdrawal. Unmodified preparations of insulin typically appear as clear substances, so they should be without particles or foreign matter. Modified preparations of insulin are typically suspensions, so they do not appear as clear substances. Check the expiration date before administering the medication. Assess the appropriateness of the drug for the patient. Review the assessment and laboratory data that may influence drug administration. Check the patient's blood glucose level, if appropriate, before administering the insulin. Verify patient name, dose, route, and time of administration.
NURSING DIAGNOSIS	Determine related factors for the nursing diagnoses based on the patient's current status. Appropriate nursing diagnoses include: • Risk for Infection • Deficient Knowledge • Risk for Injury
OUTCOME IDENTIFICATION AND PLANNING	The expected outcome to achieve when mixing two different types of medication in one syringe is the accurate withdrawal of the medication into a syringe in a sterile manner and that the proper dose is prepared.

IMPLEMENTATION

ACTION	RATIONALE
1. Gather equipment. Check medication order against the original order in the medical record, according to facility policy.	This comparison helps to identify errors that may have occurred when orders were transcribed. The primary care provider's order is the legal record of medication orders for each facility.
2. Know the actions, special nursing considerations, safe dose ranges, purpose of administration, and adverse effects of the medications to be administered. Consider the appropriateness of the medication for this patient.	This knowledge aids the nurse in evaluating the therapeutic effect of the medication in relation to the patient's disorder and can also be used to educate the patient about the medication.
3. Perform hand hygiene.	Hand hygiene prevents the spread of microorganisms.
4. Move the medication cart to the outside of the patient's room or prepare for administration in the medication area.	Organization facilitates error-free administration and saves time.
5. Unlock the medication cart or drawer. Enter pass code and scan employee identification, if required.	Locking the cart or drawer safeguards each patient's medication supply. Hospital accrediting organizations require medication carts to be locked when not in use. Entering pass code and scanning ID allows only authorized users into the system and identifies the user for documentation by the computer.
6. **Prepare medications for one patient at a time.**	This prevents errors in medication administration.
7. Read the CMAR/MAR and select the proper medications from unit stock or the patient's medication drawer.	This is the *first* check of the label.
8. Compare the labels with the CMAR/MAR. Check expiration dates and perform dosage calculations, if necessary. Scan the bar code on the package, if required.	This is the *second* check of the labels. Verify calculations with another nurse to ensure safety, if necessary.
9. If necessary, remove the cap that protects the rubber stopper on each vial.	The cap protects the rubber top.
10. **If medication is a suspension (e.g., a modified insulin, such as NPH insulin), roll and agitate the vial to mix it well.**	There is controversy regarding how to mix insulin in suspension. Some sources advise rolling the vial; others advise shaking the vial. Consult facility policy. Regardless of the method used, it is essential that the suspension be mixed well to avoid administering an inconsistent dose.
11. **Cleanse the rubber tops with antimicrobial swabs.** Allow the top to dry.	Antimicrobial swab removes surface bacterial contamination. Allowing the alcohol to dry prevents it from entering the vial on the needle.
12. Remove cap from needle by pulling it straight off. Touch the plunger only at the knob. Draw back an amount of air into the syringe that is equal to the dose of modified insulin to be withdrawn.	Pulling the cap off in a straight manner prevents accidental needlestick. Handling the plunger only by the knob ensures sterility of the shaft of the plunger. Before fluid is removed, injection of an equal amount of air is required to prevent the formation of a partial vacuum, because a vial is a sealed container. If not enough air is injected, the negative pressure makes it difficult to withdraw the medication.
13. Hold the modified vial on a flat surface. Pierce the rubber stopper in the center with the needle tip and inject the measured air into the space above the solution (Figure 1). Do not inject air into the solution. Withdraw the needle.	Unmodified insulin should never be contaminated with modified insulin. Placing air in the modified insulin first without allowing the needle to contact the insulin ensures that the second vial-entered (unmodified) insulin is not contaminated by the medication in the other vial. Air bubbled through the solution could result in withdrawal of an inaccurate amount of medication.

(*continued*)

SKILL 5 | MIXING MEDICATIONS FROM TWO VIALS IN ONE SYRINGE continued

ACTION

14. Draw back an amount of air into the syringe that is equal to the dose of unmodified insulin to be withdrawn.

15. Hold the unmodified vial on a flat surface. Pierce the rubber stopper in the center with the needle tip and inject the measured air into the space above the solution (Figure 2). Do not inject air into the solution. Keep the needle in the vial.

FIGURE 1 Injecting air into modified insulin preparation.

16. Invert the vial of unmodified insulin. Hold the vial in one hand and use the other to withdraw the medication. **Touch the plunger only at the knob. Draw up the prescribed amount of medication while holding the syringe at eye level and vertically (Figure 3).** Turn the vial over and then remove the needle from the vial.

17. Check that there are no air bubbles in the syringe.

18. **Check the amount of medication in the syringe with the medication dose and discard any surplus.**

19. **Recheck the vial label with the CMAR/MAR.**

20. Calculate the endpoint on the syringe for the combined insulin amount by adding the number of units for each dose together.

RATIONALE

A vial is a sealed container. Therefore, injection of an equal amount of air (before fluid is removed) is required to prevent the formation of a partial vacuum. If not enough air is injected, the negative pressure makes it difficult to withdraw the medication.

Air bubbled through the solution could result in withdrawal of an inaccurate amount of medication.

FIGURE 2 Injecting air into unmodified insulin vial.

Holding the syringe at eye level facilitates accurate reading, and the vertical position allows easy removal of air bubbles from the syringe. First dose is prepared and is not contaminated by insulin that contains modifiers.

The presence of air in the syringe would result in an inaccurate dose of medication.

Careful measurement ensures that correct dose is withdrawn.

This is the *third* check to ensure accuracy and to prevent errors. It must be checked now for the first medication in the syringe, as it is not possible to ensure accuracy once a second drug is in the syringe.

Allows for accurate withdrawal of the second dose.

ACTION

RATIONALE

21. Insert the needle into the modified vial and invert it, taking care not to push the plunger and inject medication from the syringe into the vial. Invert vial of modified insulin. Hold the vial in one hand and use the other to withdraw the medication. **Touch the plunger only at the knob. Draw up the prescribed amount of medication while holding the syringe at eye level and vertically (Figure 4). Take care to withdraw only the prescribed amount.** Turn the vial over and then remove the needle from the vial. Carefully recap the needle. Carefully replace the cap over the needle.

Previous addition of air eliminates need to create positive pressure. Holding the syringe at eye level facilitates accurate reading. Capping the needle prevents contamination and protects the nurse against accidental needlesticks. A one-handed recap method may be used as long as care is taken to ensure that the needle remains sterile.

FIGURE 3 Withdrawing prescribed amount of unmodified insulin.

FIGURE 4 Withdrawing modified insulin.

22. **Check the amount of medication in the syringe with the medication dose.**

Careful measurement ensures that correct dose is withdrawn.

23. **Depending on facility policy, the third check of the label may occur at this point. If so, recheck the label with the MAR before taking the medications to the patient.**

This *third* check ensures accuracy and helps to prevent errors. *Note:* Many facilities require the *third* check to occur at the bedside, after identifying the patient and before administration.

24. **Label the vials with the date and time opened, and store the vials containing the remaining medication, according to facility policy.**

Because the vial is sealed, the medication inside remains sterile and can be used for future injections. Labeling the opened vials with a date and time limits its use after a specific time period. The CDC recommends that medications packaged as multiuse vials be assigned to a single patient whenever possible (CDC, 2011).

25. Lock medication cart before leaving it.

Locking the cart or drawer safeguards the patient's medication supply. Hospital accrediting organizations require medication carts to be locked when not in use.

 26. Perform hand hygiene.

Hand hygiene deters the spread of microorganisms.

27. Proceed with administration, based on prescribed route.

See appropriate skill for prescribed route.

(continued)

SKILL 5 — MIXING MEDICATIONS FROM TWO VIALS IN ONE SYRINGE   continued

EVALUATION	The expected outcome is met when the medication is withdrawn into a syringe in a sterile manner, and the proper dose is prepared.
DOCUMENTATION *Guidelines*	It is not necessary to record the removal of the medication from the ampule. Prompt recording of administration of the medication is required immediately after it is administered.
UNEXPECTED SITUATIONS AND ASSOCIATED INTERVENTIONS	• *You contaminate the plunger before injecting air into the insulin vial:* Discard the needle and syringe and start over. *If plunger is contaminated after medication is drawn into the syringe,* it is not necessary to discard and start over. The contaminated plunger will enter the barrel of the syringe when pushing the medication out and will not contaminate the medication. • *You allow modified insulin to come in contact with the needle before entering the unmodified insulin vial:* Discard needle and syringe and start over. • *You notice that the combined amount is not the ordered amount (e.g., you have less or more units in combined syringe than ordered):* Discard syringe and start over. There is no way to know for sure which dosage is wrong or which medication should be expelled. • *You inject medication from the first vial (in syringe) into the second vial:* Discard vial and syringe and start over.
SPECIAL CONSIDERATIONS *General Considerations*	• A patient with diabetes who is visually impaired may find it helpful to use a magnifying apparatus that fits around the syringe. • Before attempting to explain or demonstrate devices that help low-vision diabetic patients to prepare their medication, attempt to use the device yourself under similar circumstances. To detect any difficulties the patient may experience, practice using the aid with your eyes closed or in a poorly lit room.
Infant and Child Considerations	School-age children are generally able to prepare and administer their own injections, such as insulin, with supervision (Kyle & Carman, 2013). Parents/significant others and the child should be involved in teaching.

SKILL 6 — ADMINISTERING AN INTRADERMAL INJECTION

Intradermal injections are administered into the dermis, just below the epidermis. The intradermal route has the longest absorption time of all parenteral routes. For this reason, intradermal injections are used for sensitivity tests, such as tuberculin and allergy tests, and local anesthesia. The advantage of the intradermal route for these tests is that the body's reaction to substances is easily visible, and degrees of reaction are discernible by comparative study.

Sites commonly used are the inner surface of the forearm and the upper back, under the scapula. Equipment used for an intradermal injection includes a tuberculin syringe calibrated in tenths and hundredths of a milliliter and a 0.25- to 0.5-inch, 25- or 27-gauge needle. The dosage given intradermally is small, usually less than 0.5 mL. The angle of administration for an intradermal injection is 5 to 15 degrees.

DELEGATION CONSIDERATIONS	The administration of an intradermal injection is not delegated to nursing assistive personnel (NAP) or to unlicensed assistive personnel (UAP). Depending on the state's nurse practice act and the organization's policies and procedures, the administration of an intradermal injection may be delegated to licensed practical/vocational nurses (LPN/LVNs). The decision to delegate must be based on careful analysis of the patient's needs and circumstances, as well as the qualifications of the person to whom the task is being delegated.

EQUIPMENT	
• Prescribed medication • Sterile syringe, usually a tuberculin syringe calibrated in tenths and hundredths, and a needle, ¼- to ½-inch, 25- or 27-gauge • Antimicrobial swab • Disposable gloves	• Small gauze square • Computer-generated Medication Administration Record (CMAR) or Medication Administration Record (MAR) • PPE, as indicated

---

ASSESSMENT

Assess the patient for any allergies. Check expiration date before administering medication. Assess the appropriateness of the drug for the patient. Review assessment and laboratory data that may influence drug administration. Assess the site on the patient where the injection is to be given. Avoid areas of broken or open skin. Avoid areas that are highly pigmented, and those that have lesions, bruises, or scars and are hairy. Assess the patient's knowledge of the medication. This may provide an opportune time for patient education. Verify the patient's name, dose, route, and time of administration.

NURSING DIAGNOSIS

Determine related factors for the nursing diagnoses based on the patient's current status. Appropriate nursing diagnoses may include:

- Deficient Knowledge
- Risk for Infection
- Risk for Injury

OUTCOME IDENTIFICATION AND PLANNING

The expected outcome to achieve when administering an intradermal injection is the appearance of a wheal at the injection site. Other outcomes that may be appropriate include the following: the patient refrains from rubbing the site; the patient's anxiety is decreased; the patient does not experience adverse effects; and the patient understands and complies with the medication regimen.

IMPLEMENTATION

ACTION	RATIONALE
1. Gather equipment. Check each medication order against the original order in the medical record according to facility policy. Clarify any inconsistencies. Check the patient's chart for allergies.	This comparison helps to identify errors that may have occurred when orders were transcribed. The primary care provider's order is the legal record of medication orders for each facility.
2. Know the actions, special nursing considerations, safe dose ranges, purpose of administration, and adverse effects of the medications to be administered. Consider the appropriateness of the medication for this patient.	This knowledge aids the nurse in evaluating the therapeutic effect of the medication in relation to the patient's disorder and can also be used to educate the patient about the medication.
3. Perform hand hygiene.	Hand hygiene deters the spread of microorganisms.
4. Move the medication cart to the outside of the patient's room or prepare for administration in the medication area.	Organization facilitates error-free administration and saves time.
5. Unlock the medication cart or drawer. Enter pass code and scan employee identification, if required.	Locking the cart or drawer safeguards each patient's medication supply. Hospital accrediting organizations require medication carts to be locked when not in use. Entering pass code and scanning ID allows only authorized users into the system and identifies the user for documentation by the computer.
6. Prepare medications for one patient at a time.	This prevents errors in medication administration.
7. Read the CMAR/MAR and select the proper medication from unit stock or the patient's medication drawer.	This is the *first* check of the label.

(continued)

SKILL 6 ADMINISTERING AN INTRADERMAL INJECTION continued

ACTION	RATIONALE
8. Compare the label with the CMAR/MAR. Check expiration dates and perform calculations, if necessary. Scan the bar code on the package, if required.	This is the *second* check of the label. Verify calculations with another nurse to ensure safety.
9. If necessary, withdraw the medication from an ampule or vial as described in Skills 3 and 4.	
10. **Depending on facility policy, the third check of the label may occur at this point. If so, when all medications for one patient have been prepared, recheck the labels with the CMAR/MAR before taking the medications to the patient.**	This *third* check ensures accuracy and helps to prevent errors. *Note:* Many facilities require the *third* check to occur at the bedside, after identifying the patient and before administration.
11. Lock the medication cart before leaving it.	Locking the cart or drawer safeguards the patient's medication supply. Hospital accrediting organizations require medication carts to be locked when not in use.
12. Transport medications to the patient's bedside carefully, and keep the medications in sight at all times.	Careful handling and close observation prevent accidental or deliberate disarrangement of medications.
13. **Ensure that the patient receives the medications at the correct time.**	Check agency policy, which may allow for administration within a period of 30 minutes before or 30 minutes after the designated time.
14. Perform hand hygiene and put on PPE, if indicated.	Hand hygiene and PPE prevent the spread of microorganisms. PPE is required based on transmission precautions.
15. **Identify the patient. Compare the information with the CMAR/MAR. The patient should be identified using at least two methods** (The Joint Commission, 2013):	Identifying the patient ensures the right patient receives the medications and helps prevent errors. The patient's room number or physical location is not used as an identifier (The Joint Commission, 2013). Replace the identification band if it is missing or inaccurate in any way.
a. Check the name on the patient's identification band.	
b. Check the identification number on the patient's identification band.	
c. Check the birth date on the patient's identification band.	
d. Ask the patient to state his or her name and birth date, based on facility policy.	This requires a response from the patient, but illness and strange surroundings often cause patients to be confused.
16. Close the door to the room or pull the bedside curtain.	This provides patient privacy.
17. **Complete necessary assessments before administering medications. Check allergy bracelet or ask the patient about allergies. Explain the purpose and action of the medication to the patient.**	Assessment is a prerequisite to administration of medications. Explanation provides rationale, increases knowledge, and reduces anxiety.
18. Scan the patient's bar code on the identification band, if required.	Provides an additional check to ensure that the medication is given to the right patient.
19. **Based on facility policy, the third check of the label may occur at this point. If so, recheck the labels with the CMAR/MAR before administering the medications to the patient.**	Many facilities require the *third* check to occur at the bedside, after identifying the patient and before administration. If facility policy directs the *third* check at this time, this *third* check ensures accuracy and helps to prevent errors.
20. Put on clean gloves.	Gloves help prevent exposure to contaminants.
21. Select an appropriate administration site. Assist the patient to the appropriate position for the site chosen. Drape, as needed, to expose only site area to be used.	Appropriate site prevents injury and allows for accurate reading of the test site at the appropriate time. Draping provides privacy and warmth.
22. Cleanse the site with an antimicrobial swab while wiping with a firm, circular motion and moving outward from the injection site. Allow the skin to dry.	Pathogens on the skin can be forced into the tissues by the needle. Moving from the center outward prevents contamination of the site. Allowing skin to dry prevents introducing alcohol into the tissue, which can be irritating and uncomfortable.

ACTION	RATIONALE
23. Remove the needle cap with the nondominant hand by pulling it straight off.	This technique lessens the risk of an accidental needlestick.
24. Use the nondominant hand to spread the skin taut over the injection site (Figure 1).	Taut skin provides an easy entrance into intradermal tissue.
25. Hold the syringe in the dominant hand, between the thumb and forefinger with the bevel of the needle up.	Using the dominant hand allows for easy, appropriate handling of the syringe. Having the bevel up allows for smooth piercing of the skin and introduction of medication into the dermis.
26. Hold the syringe at a 5- to 15-degree angle from the site. Place the needle almost flat against the patient's skin (Figure 2), bevel side up, and insert the needle into the skin. Insert the needle only about ⅛ inch with entire bevel under the skin.	The dermis is entered when the needle is held as nearly parallel to the skin as possible and is inserted about ⅛ inch.

FIGURE 1 Spreading skin taut over injection site.

FIGURE 2 Inserting needle almost level with skin.

ACTION	RATIONALE
27. Once the needle is in place, steady the lower end of the syringe. Slide your dominant hand to the end of the plunger.	Prevents injury and inadvertent advancement or withdrawal of needle.
28. Slowly inject the agent while watching for a small wheal or blister to appear (Figure 3).	The appearance of a wheal indicates the medication is in the dermis.

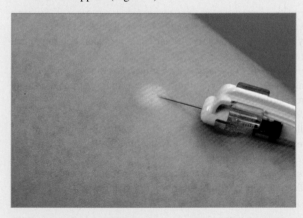

FIGURE 3 Observing for wheal while injecting medication.

ACTION	RATIONALE
29. Withdraw the needle quickly at the same angle that it was inserted. Do not recap the used needle. Engage the safety shield or needle guard.	Withdrawing the needle quickly and at the angle at which it entered the skin minimizes tissue damage and discomfort for the patient. Safety shield or needle guard prevents accidental needlestick injury.
30. **Do not massage the area after removing needle. Tell the patient not to rub or scratch the site. If necessary, gently blot the site with a dry gauze square. Do not apply pressure or rub the site.**	Massaging the area where an intradermal injection is given may spread the medication to underlying subcutaneous tissue.

(continued)

SKILL 6 ADMINISTERING AN INTRADERMAL INJECTION continued

ACTION	RATIONALE
31. Assist the patient to a position of comfort.	This provides for the well-being of the patient.
32. Discard the needle and syringe in the appropriate receptacle.	Proper disposal of the needle prevents injury.
33. Remove gloves and additional PPE, if used. Perform hand hygiene.	Removing PPE properly reduces the risk for infection transmission and contamination of other items. Hand hygiene prevents the spread of microorganisms.
34. Document the administration of the medication immediately after administration. See Documentation section below.	Timely documentation helps to ensure patient safety.
35. Evaluate the patient's response to the medication within the appropriate time frame.	The patient needs to be evaluated for therapeutic and adverse effects from the medication.
36. Observe the area for signs of a reaction at determined intervals after administration. Inform the patient of the need for inspection.	With many intradermal injections, you need to look for a localized reaction in the area of the injection at the appropriate interval(s) determined by the type of medication and purpose. Explaining this to the patient increases compliance.

EVALUATION

The expected outcomes are met when you note a wheal at the injection site; the patient refrains from rubbing the site; the patient's anxiety is decreased; the patient did not experience adverse effects; and the patient verbalizes an understanding of, and complies with, the medication regimen.

DOCUMENTATION

Guidelines

Record each medication administered on the CMAR/MAR or record using the required format, including date, time, and the site of administration, immediately after administration. Some facilities recommend circling the injection site with ink. Circling the injection site easily identifies the intradermal injection site and allows for future careful observation of the exact area. If using a bar-code system, medication administration is automatically recorded when the bar code is scanned. PRN medications require documentation of the reason for administration. Prompt recording avoids the possibility of accidentally repeating the administration of the drug. If the drug was refused or omitted, record this in the appropriate area on the medication record and notify the primary care provider. This verifies the reason medication was omitted and ensures that the primary care provider is aware of the patient's condition.

UNEXPECTED SITUATIONS AND ASSOCIATED INTERVENTIONS

- *You do not note a wheal or blister at the injection site:* Medication has been injected subcutaneously. Document according to facility policy and inform the primary care provider. You may need to obtain an order to repeat the procedure.
- *Medication leaks out of the injection site before the needle is withdrawn:* Needle was inserted less than ⅛ inch. Document according to facility policy and inform the primary care provider. You may need to obtain an order to repeat the procedure.
- *You stick yourself with the needle before injection:* Discard needle and syringe appropriately. Follow facility policy regarding needlestick injury. Prepare new syringe with medication and administer to patient. Complete appropriate paperwork and follow facility's policy regarding accidental needlestick injuries.
- *You stick yourself with the needle after injection:* Discard needle and syringe appropriately. Follow facility policy regarding needlestick injury. Complete appropriate paperwork and follow facility's policy regarding accidental needlesticks.

SPECIAL CONSIDERATIONS

- Ongoing assessment is an important part of nursing care for both evaluation of patient response to administered medications and early detection of adverse effects. If an adverse effect is suspected, withhold further medication doses and notify the patient's primary care provider. Additional intervention is based on type of reaction and patient assessment.
- Aspiration, pulling back on the plunger after insertion and before administration, is not recommended for an intradermal injection. The dermis does not contain large blood vessels.
- Some agencies recommend administering intradermal injections with the bevel down instead of the bevel up. Check facility policy.

SKILL 7 ADMINISTERING A SUBCUTANEOUS INJECTION

Subcutaneous injections are administered into the adipose tissue layer just below the epidermis and dermis. This tissue has few blood vessels, so drugs administered here have a slow, sustained rate of absorption into the capillaries.

It is important to choose the right equipment to ensure depositing the medication into the intended tissue layer and not the underlying muscle. Equipment used for a subcutaneous injection includes a syringe of appropriate volume for the amount of drug being administered. An insulin injection pen may be used for subcutaneous injection of insulin (see the accompanying Skill Variation for technique). A 25- to 30-gauge, ⅜- to 1-inch needle can be used; ⅜- and ⅝-inch needles are most commonly used for subcutaneous injections. Choose the needle length based on the amount of subcutaneous tissue present, which is based on the patient's body weight and build (Annersten & Willman, 2005). Some medications are packaged in prefilled cartridges with a needle attached. Confirm that the provided needle is appropriate for the patient before use. If not, the medication will have to be transferred to another syringe and the appropriate needle attached.

Review the specifics of the particular medication before administrating it to the patient. Various sites may be used for subcutaneous injections, including the outer aspect of the upper arm, the abdomen (from below the costal margin to the iliac crests), the anterior aspects of the thigh, the upper back, and the upper ventral gluteal area. Figure 1 displays the sites on the body where subcutaneous injections can be given. Absorption rates differ at different sites. Injections in the abdomen are absorbed most rapidly; ones in the arms are absorbed somewhat more slowly; those in the thighs, even more slowly; and those in the upper ventral or dorsogluteal areas have the slowest absorption (American Diabetes Association [ADA], 2004).

FIGURE 1 Body sites where subcutaneous injections can be given.

Subcutaneous injections are administered at a 45- to 90-degree angle. Choose the angle of needle insertion based on the amount of subcutaneous tissue present and the length of the needle. Generally, insert the shorter, ⅜-inch needle, at a 90-degree angle and the longer, ⅝-inch needle, at a 45-degree angle.

Recommendations differ regarding pinching or bunching a skin fold for administration. Pinching is advised for thinner patients and when a longer needle is used, to lift the adipose tissue away from underlying muscle and tissue. If pinching is used, once the needle is inserted, release the skin to avoid injecting into the compressed tissue.

(continued)

SKILL 7 ADMINISTERING A SUBCUTANEOUS INJECTION continued

Aspiration, or pulling back on the plunger to check that a blood vessel has been entered, is not necessary and has not proved to be a reliable indicator of needle placement. The likelihood of injecting into a blood vessel is small (Crawford & Johnson, 2012). The American Diabetes Association (2004) has stated that routine aspiration is not necessary when injecting insulin. **Aspiration is definitely contraindicated with administration of heparin because this action can result in hematoma formation.**

Usually, no more than 1 mL of solution is given subcutaneously. Giving larger amounts adds to the patient's discomfort and may predispose to poor absorption. It is necessary to rotate sites or areas for injection if the patient is to receive frequent injections. This helps to prevent buildup of fibrous tissue and permits complete absorption of the medication.

Box 7-1 discusses techniques for reducing discomfort when injecting medications subcutaneously or intramuscularly.

BOX 7-1 REDUCING DISCOMFORT IN SUBCUTANEOUS AND INTRAMUSCULAR ADMINISTRATIONS

The following are recommended techniques for reducing discomfort when injecting medications subcutaneously or intramuscularly:

- Select a needle of the smallest gauge that is appropriate for the site and solution to be injected, and select the correct needle length.
- Be sure the needle is free of medication that may irritate superficial tissues as the needle is inserted. The recommended procedure is to use two needles—one to remove the medication from the vial or ampule and a second one to inject the medication. If medication is in a prefilled syringe with a non-removable needle and has dripped back on the needle during preparation, gently tap the barrel to remove the excess solution.
- Use the Z-track technique for intramuscular injections to prevent leakage of medication into the needle track, thus minimizing discomfort.
- Inject the medication into relaxed muscles. More pressure and discomfort occur when the medication is injected into a contracted muscle.

- Do not inject areas that feel hard on palpation or tender to the patient.
- Insert the needle with a dart-like motion without hesitation, and remove it quickly at the same angle at which it was inserted. These techniques reduce discomfort and tissue irritation.
- Do not administer more solution in one injection than is recommended for the site. Injecting more solution creates excess pressure in the area and increases discomfort.
- Inject the solution slowly so that it may be dispersed more easily into the surrounding tissue (10 seconds per 1 mL).
- Apply gentle pressure after injection, unless this technique is contraindicated.
- Allow the patient who is fearful of injections to talk about his or her fears. Answer the patient's questions truthfully, and explain the nature and purpose of the injection. Taking the time to offer support often allays fears and decreases discomfort.
- Rotate sites when the patient is to receive repeated injections. Injections in the same site may cause undue discomfort, irritation, or abscesses in tissues.

DELEGATION CONSIDERATIONS	The administration of a subcutaneous injection is not delegated to nursing assistive personnel (NAP) or to unlicensed assistive personnel (UAP). Depending on the state's nurse practice act and the organization's policies and procedures, the administration of a subcutaneous injection may be delegated to licensed practical/vocational nurses (LPN/LVNs). The decision to delegate must be based on careful analysis of the patient's needs and circumstances, as well as the qualifications of the person to whom the task is being delegated.
EQUIPMENT	• Prescribed medication • Sterile syringe and needle. Needle size depends on the medication to be administered and patient body type (see previous discussion). • Antimicrobial swab • Non-latex, disposable gloves • Small gauze square • Computer-generated Medication Administration Record (CMAR) or Medication Administration Record (MAR) • PPE, as indicated

ASSESSMENT

Assess the patient for any allergies. Check expiration date before administering medication. Assess the appropriateness of the drug for the patient. Verify patient name, dose, route, and time of administration. Review assessment and laboratory data that may influence drug administration. Assess the site on the patient where the injection is to be given. Avoid sites that are bruised, tender, hard, swollen, inflamed, or scarred. These conditions could affect absorption or cause discomfort and injury (Hunter, 2008). Assess the patient's knowledge of the medication. If the patient has deficient knowledge about the medication, this may be the appropriate time to begin education about it. If the medication may affect the patient's vital signs, assess them before administration. If the medication is for pain relief, assess the patient's pain before and after administration.

NURSING DIAGNOSIS

Determine related factors for the nursing diagnoses based on the patient's current status. Appropriate nursing diagnoses may include:

- Deficient Knowledge
- Acute Pain
- Risk for Injury

OUTCOME IDENTIFICATION AND PLANNING

The expected outcome is that the patient receives the medication via the subcutaneous route. Other outcomes that may be appropriate include the following: the patient's anxiety is decreased; the patient does not experience adverse effects; and the patient understands and complies with the medication regimen.

IMPLEMENTATION

ACTION	RATIONALE
1. Gather equipment. Check each medication order against the original order in the medical record, according to facility policy. Clarify any inconsistencies. Check the patient's chart for allergies.	This comparison helps to identify errors that may have occurred when orders were transcribed. The primary care provider's order is the legal record of medication orders for each facility.
2. Know the actions, special nursing considerations, safe dose ranges, purpose of administration, and adverse effects of the medications to be administered. Consider the appropriateness of the medication for this patient.	This knowledge aids the nurse in evaluating the therapeutic effect of the medication in relation to the patient's disorder and can also be used to educate the patient about the medication.
3. Perform hand hygiene.	Hand hygiene prevents the spread of microorganisms.
4. Move the medication cart to the outside of the patient's room or prepare for administration in the medication area.	Organization facilitates error-free administration and saves time.
5. Unlock the medication cart or drawer. Enter pass code and scan employee identification, if required.	Locking the cart or drawer safeguards each patient's medication supply. Hospital accrediting organizations require medication carts to be locked when not in use. Entering pass code and scanning ID allows only authorized users into the computer system and identifies the user for documentation by the computer.
6. **Prepare medications for one patient at a time.**	This prevents errors in medication administration.
7. Read the CMAR/MAR and select the proper medication from unit stock or the patient's medication drawer.	This is the *first* check of the label.
8. Compare the label with the CMAR/MAR. Check expiration dates and perform calculations, if necessary. Scan the bar code on the package, if required.	This is the *second* check of the label. Verify calculations with another nurse to ensure safety, if necessary.
9. If necessary, withdraw medication from an ampule or vial as described in Skills 3 and 4.	

(continued)

SKILL 7 ADMINISTERING A SUBCUTANEOUS INJECTION continued

ACTION	RATIONALE

10. **Depending on facility policy, the third check of the label may occur at this point. If so, when all medications for one patient have been prepared, recheck the labels with the CMAR/MAR before taking the medications to the patient.**

This *third* check ensures accuracy and helps to prevent errors. *Note:* Many facilities require the *third* check to occur at the bedside, after identifying the patient and before administration.

11. Lock the medication cart before leaving it.

Locking the cart or drawer safeguards the patient's medication supply. Hospital accrediting organizations require medication carts to be locked when not in use.

12. Transport medications to the patient's bedside carefully, and keep the medications in sight at all times.

Careful handling and close observation prevent accidental or deliberate disarrangement of medications.

13. **Ensure that the patient receives the medications at the correct time.**

Check agency policy, which may allow for administration within a period of 30 minutes before or 30 minutes after the designated time.

14. Perform hand hygiene and put on PPE, if indicated.

Hand hygiene and PPE prevent the spread of microorganisms. PPE is required based on transmission precautions.

15. **Identify the patient. Compare the information with the CMAR/MAR. The patient should be identified using at least two methods** (The Joint Commission, 2013):

Identifying the patient ensures the right patient receives the medications and helps prevent errors. The patient's room number or physical location is not used as an identifier (The Joint Commission, 2013). Replace the identification band if it is missing or inaccurate in any way.

a. Check the name on the patient's identification band.

b. Check the identification number on the patient's identification band.

c. Check the birth date on the patient's identification band.

d. Ask the patient to state his or her name and birth date, based on facility policy.

This requires a response from the patient, but illness and strange surroundings often cause patients to be confused.

16. Close the door to the room or pull the bedside curtain.

This provides patient privacy.

17. **Complete necessary assessments before administering medications. Check the patient's allergy bracelet or ask the patient about allergies. Explain the purpose and action of the medication to the patient.**

Assessment is a prerequisite to administration of medications. Explanation provides rationale, increases knowledge, and reduces anxiety.

18. Scan the patient's bar code on the identification band, if required (Figure 2).

Scanning provides an additional check to ensure that the medication is given to the right patient.

FIGURE 2 Scanning bar code on the patient's identification bracelet. *(Photo by B. Proud.)*

19. **Based on facility policy, the third check of the label may occur at this point. If so, recheck the labels with the CMAR/MAR before administering the medications to the patient.**

Many facilities require the *third* check to occur at the bedside, after identifying the patient and before administration. If facility policy directs the *third* check at this time, this *third* check ensures accuracy and helps to prevent errors.

ACTION	RATIONALE
20. Put on clean gloves.	Gloves help prevent exposure to contaminants.
21. Select an appropriate administration site.	Appropriate site prevents injury and allows for accurate reading of the test site at the appropriate time.
22. Assist the patient to the appropriate position for the site chosen. Drape, as needed, to expose only site area to be used.	Appropriate site prevents injury. Draping helps maintain the patient's privacy.
23. Identify the appropriate landmarks for the site chosen.	Good visualization is necessary to establish the correct site location and to avoid tissue damage.
24. Cleanse the area around the injection site with an antimicrobial swab. Use a firm, circular motion while moving outward from the injection site (Figure 3). Allow the area to dry.	Pathogens on the skin can be forced into the tissues by the needle. Moving from the center outward prevents contamination of the site. Allowing skin to dry prevents introducing alcohol into the tissue, which can be irritating and uncomfortable.
25. Remove the needle cap with the nondominant hand, pulling it straight off.	The cap protects the needle from contact with microorganisms. This technique lessens the risk of an accidental needlestick.
26. Grasp and bunch the area surrounding the injection site or spread the skin taut at the site (Figure 4).	Decision to create a skin fold is based on the nurse's assessment of the patient and needle length used. Pinching is advised for thinner patients and when a longer needle is used, to lift the adipose tissue away from underlying muscle and tissue. If pinching is used, once the needle is inserted, release the skin to avoid injecting into compressed tissue. If skin is pulled taut, it provides easy, less painful entry into the subcutaneous tissue.

FIGURE 3 Cleaning injection site.

FIGURE 4 Bunching tissue at injection site.

27. Hold the syringe in the dominant hand between the thumb and forefinger. Inject the needle quickly at a 45- to 90-degree angle (Figure 5).	Inserting the needle quickly causes less pain to the patient. Subcutaneous tissue is abundant in well-nourished, well-hydrated people and spare in emaciated, dehydrated, or very thin persons. For a person with little subcutaneous tissue, it is best to insert the needle at a 45-degree angle.

FIGURE 5 Inserting needle.

(*continued*)

SKILL 7

ADMINISTERING A SUBCUTANEOUS INJECTION continued

ACTION	RATIONALE
28. After the needle is in place, release the tissue. If you have a large skin fold pinched up, ensure that the needle stays in place as the skin is released. Immediately move your non-dominant hand to steady the lower end of the syringe. Slide your dominant hand to the end of the plunger. Avoid moving the syringe.	Injecting the solution into compressed tissues results in pressure against nerve fibers and creates discomfort. If there is a large skin fold, the skin may retract away from the needle. The non-dominant hand secures the syringe. Moving the syringe could cause damage to the tissues and inadvertent administration into an incorrect area.
29. Inject the medication slowly (at a rate of 10 sec/mL).	Rapid injection of the solution creates pressure in the tissues, resulting in discomfort.
30. Withdraw the needle quickly at the same angle at which it was inserted, while supporting the surrounding tissue with your nondominant hand.	Slow withdrawal of the needle pulls the tissues and causes discomfort. Applying counter traction around the injection site helps to prevent pulling on the tissue as the needle is withdrawn. Removing the needle at the same angle at which it was inserted minimizes tissue damage and discomfort for the patient.
31. Using a gauze square, apply gentle pressure to the site after the needle is withdrawn (Figure 6). **Do not massage the site.**	Massaging the site can damage underlying tissue and increase the absorption of the medication. Massaging after heparin administration can contribute to hematoma formation. Massaging after an insulin injection may contribute to unpredictable absorption of the medication.

FIGURE 6 Applying pressure to injection site.

ACTION	RATIONALE
32. Do not recap the used needle. Engage the safety shield or needle guard. Discard the needle and syringe in the appropriate receptacle.	Safety shield or needle guard prevents accidental needlestick. Proper disposal of the needle prevents injury.
33. Assist the patient to a position of comfort.	This provides for the well-being of the patient.
34. Remove gloves and additional PPE, if used. Perform hand hygiene.	Removing PPE properly reduces the risk for infection transmission and contamination of other items. Hand hygiene prevents the spread of microorganisms.
35. Document the administration of the medication immediately after administration. See Documentation section on page 37.	Timely documentation helps to ensure patient safety.
36. Evaluate the patient's response to the medication within the appropriate time frame for the particular medication.	The patient needs to be evaluated for therapeutic and adverse effects from the medication.

EVALUATION

The expected outcomes are met when the patient receives the medication via the subcutaneous route; the patient's anxiety is decreased; the patient does not experience adverse effects; and the patient understands and complies with the medication regimen.

DOCUMENTATION

Guidelines

Record each medication given on the CMAR/MAR or record using the required format, including date, dose, time, and the site of administration, immediately after administration. If using a bar-code system, medication administration is automatically recorded when the bar code is scanned. PRN medications require documentation of the reason for administration. Prompt recording avoids the possibility of accidentally repeating the administration of the drug. If the drug was refused or omitted, record this in the appropriate area on the medication record and notify the primary care provider. This verifies the reason medication was omitted and ensures that the primary care provider is aware of the patient's condition.

UNEXPECTED SITUATIONS AND ASSOCIATED INTERVENTIONS

- *When skin fold is released, needle pulls out of skin:* Engage safety shield or needle guard. Appropriately discard needle. Attach new needle to syringe and administer injection.
- *Patient refuses to let you administer medication in a different location:* Explain the rationale behind rotating injection sites. Discuss other available injection sites with the patient. If the patient will still not allow injection in another area, administer medication to patient, document patient's refusal of rotation of injection site and discussion, and notify primary care provider.
- *You stick yourself with the needle before injection:* Discard needle and syringe appropriately. Follow facility policy regarding needlestick injury. Prepare new syringe with medication and administer to patient. Complete appropriate paperwork and follow facility's policy regarding accidental needlestick injuries.
- *You stick yourself with the needle after injection:* Discard needle and syringe appropriately. Complete appropriate paperwork and follow facility's policy regarding accidental needlestick injuries.
- *During injection, patient pulls away from the needle before the medication is delivered fully:* Remove and appropriately discard needle. Attach a new needle to syringe and administer remaining medication at a different site. Document events and interventions according to facility policy.

SPECIAL CONSIDERATIONS

General Considerations

- Ongoing assessment is an important part of nursing care for both evaluation of patient response to administered medications and early detection of adverse effects. If an adverse effect is suspected, withhold further medication doses and notify the patient's primary care provider. Additional intervention is based on type of reaction and patient assessment.
- Heparin is administered subcutaneously. The abdomen is the most commonly used administration site. Avoid the area 2 inches around the umbilicus and the belt line. The manufacturer's directions for subcutaneous administration of low–molecular-weight heparin preparations, such as enoxaparin (Lovenox), include specific instructions regarding administration site and technique (Sanofi Aventis, 2012). Administer enoxaparin in an area on the abdomen between the left or right anterolateral and left or right posterolateral abdominal wall (Figure 7). To administer the medication, pinch the tissue gently and insert the needle at a 90-degree angle. In addition, enoxaparin is packaged in a prefilled syringe with an air bubble. Do not expel the air bubble before administration.

Anterior view   Posterior view

FIGURE 7 Sites for administration of enoxaparin.

Infant and Child Considerations

- Do not tell a child that an injection will not hurt. Describe the feel of the injection as a pinch or a sting. A child who believes you have been dishonest with him/her is less likely to cooperate with future procedures.

Older Adult Considerations

- Many older patients have less adipose tissue. Adjust the needle length and insertion angle accordingly. (Refer to discussion earlier in Skill.) You do not want to inadvertently give a subcutaneous medication intramuscularly.

(continued)

SKILL 7 ADMINISTERING A SUBCUTANEOUS INJECTION continued

Home Care Considerations

- Reuse of syringes in the home setting is not recommended.
- Because absorption rates vary from site to site, it is recommended that patients administering their own insulin use the same area of the body at the same time every day to ensure more consistent absorption and prevent tissue changes from repeated use of the same site (Ashenbrenner & Veneble, 2012; ADA, 2004). Rotate injection sites within the area of the body being used.
- Changes and improvements to insulin syringes to make injections painless have resulted in thinner, shorter, sharper, and better lubricated needles. As a result, after one injection the tip of the fine needles can bend and form a hook that can tear tissue if reused. In addition, these fine needles can break and leave fragments in the skin and tissue if reused. Reuse results in more painful injections related to a reduction in needle lubricant and tip damage. Therefore, teach patients to use a new needle and syringe for each injection.
- Encourage patients to consult the policies of their local government regarding contaminated and sharps waste disposal. Teach patients to dispose of needles and syringes in a hard, plastic container. Liquid detergent or liquid fabric softener containers are good choices. Never use glass containers.

SKILL VARIATION — Using an Insulin Injection Pen to Administer Insulin via the Subcutaneous Route

Prepare medication as outlined in steps 1–13 above (Skill 7).

1. Perform hand hygiene and put on PPE, as indicated.

2. Identify the patient.

3. Explain the procedure to patient.
4. Close the door to the room or pull the bedside curtain.
5. **Complete necessary assessments before administering medications. Check the patient's allergy bracelet or ask the patient about allergies. Explain the purpose and action of the medication to the patient.**
6. Scan the patient's bar code on the identification band, if required.
7. **Based on facility policy, the third check of the label may occur at this point. If so, recheck the labels with the CMAR/ MAR before administering the medications to the patient.**
8. Select an appropriate administration site.
9. Assist the patient to the appropriate position for the site chosen. Drape, as needed, to expose only area of site to be used.
10. Identify the appropriate landmarks for the site chosen.
11. Remove the pen cap.
12. Insert an insulin cartridge into the pen, if necessary, following the manufacturer's directions.
13. Clean the tip of the reservoir with alcohol.
14. Invert the pen 20 times to mix if using an insulin suspension.
15. Remove the protective tab from the needle.
16. Screw the needle onto the reservoir.
17. Remove the outer and inner needle caps.
18. Hold the pen upright and tap to force any air bubbles to the top.
19. Dial the dose selector to 2 units to perform an "air shot" to get rid of bubbles.
20. Hold the pen upright and press the plunger firmly. Watch for a drop of insulin at the needle tip.

FIGURE A Patient using insulin pen. *(Photo by B. Proud.)*

21. Check the drug reservoir to make sure sufficient insulin is available for the dose.
22. Check that the dose selector is at "0," then dial the units of insulin for the dose.
23. Put on gloves.
24. Clean the injection site and administer the subcutaneous injection, holding the pen like a dart. Push the button on the pen all the way in (Figure A).
25. Keep the button depressed and count to 6 before removing from the skin.
26. Remove the needle from the pen and dispose in a sharps container.
27. Remove gloves and additional PPE, if used.

28. Perform hand hygiene.

29. Document administration on the CMAR/MAR, including the injection site.

(Adapted from Moshang, J. (2005). Making a point about insulin pens. *Nursing, 35*(2), 46–47.)

SKILL 8 | ADMINISTERING AN INTRAMUSCULAR INJECTION

Intramuscular injections deliver medication through the skin and subcutaneous tissues into certain muscles. Muscles have a larger and a greater number of blood vessels than subcutaneous tissue, allowing faster onset of action than with subcutaneous injections. An intramuscular injection is chosen when a reasonably rapid systemic uptake of the drug is needed by the body and when a relatively prolonged action is required. Some medications administered intramuscularly are formulated to have a longer duration of effect. The deposit of medication creates a depot at the injection site, designed to deliver slow, sustained release over hours, days, or weeks.

To administer an intramuscular injection correctly and effectively, choose the right equipment, select the appropriate location, use the correct technique, and deliver the correct dose. Inject the medication into the denser part of the muscle fascia below the subcutaneous tissues. This is ideal because skeletal muscles have fewer pain-sensing nerves than subcutaneous tissue and can absorb larger volumes of solution because of the rapid uptake of the drug into the bloodstream via the muscle fibers (Hunter, 2008).

It is important to choose the right needle length for a particular intramuscular injection. Needle length should be based on the site for injection and the patient's age. (See Table 8-1 for intramuscular needle length recommendations.) Patients who are obese may require a longer needle, and emaciated patients may require a shorter needle. Appropriate gauge is determined by the medication being administered. Generally, biologic agents and medications in aqueous solutions should be administered with a 20- to 25-gauge needle. Medications in oil-based solutions should be administered with an 18- to 25-gauge needle. Many medications come in prefilled syringe units. If a needle is provided on the prefilled unit, ensure that the needle on the unit is the appropriate length for the patient and situation.

Table 8-1 INTRAMUSCULAR INJECTION NEEDLE LENGTH	
SITE/AGE	NEEDLE LENGTH
Vastus lateralis	⅝″ to 1¼″
Deltoid (children)	⅝″ to 1¼″
Deltoid (adults)	1″ to 1½″
Ventrogluteal (adults)	1½″

Note: Patients who are obese may require a longer needle (Zaybak et al., 2007) and those who are emaciated may require a shorter needle. (Adapted from Centers for Disease Control and Prevention (CDC). (2012). *The pink book: Appendices. Epidemiology and prevention of vaccine preventable diseases* (11th ed.). Appendix D. Vaccine administration. Vaccine administration guidelines. Available www.cdc.gov/vaccines/pubs/pinkbook/pinkappendx.htm#appd; Centers for Disease Control and Prevention (CDC). (2008). *Needle length and injection site of intramuscular injections.* Available http://www.cdc.gov/vaccines/ed/encounter08/Downloads/Table7.pdf; and Nicoll, L., & Hesby, A. (2002). Intramuscular injection: An integrative research review and guideline for evidence-based practice. *Applied Nursing Research, 16*(2), 149–162.)

To avoid complications, be able to identify anatomic landmarks and site boundaries. See Figure 1 for a depiction of anatomic landmarks and site boundaries for potential intramuscular injection sites. Consider the age of the patient, medication type, and medication volume when selecting an intramuscular injection site. (See Table 8-2 for information related to intramuscular site selection.) Rotate the sites used to administer intramuscular medications when therapy requires repeated injections. Whatever pattern of rotating sites is used, a description of it should appear in the patient's plan of nursing care. Depending on the site selected, it may be necessary to reposition the patient (see Table 8-3).

Use accurate, careful technique when administering intramuscular injections. If care is not taken, possible complications include abscesses; cellulites; injury to blood vessels, bones, and nerves; lingering pain; tissue necrosis; and periostitis (inflammation of the membrane covering a bone). Administer the intramuscular injection so that the needle is perpendicular to the patient's body. This ensures it is given using an injection angle between 72 and 90 degrees (Katsma & Katsma, 2000).

(continued)

SKILL 8 ADMINISTERING AN INTRAMUSCULAR INJECTION continued

FIGURE 1 Sites for intramuscular injections. Descriptions for locating sites are given in the text. (**A**) Ventrogluteal site is located by placing palm on greater trochanter and index finger toward the anterosuperior iliac spine. (**B**) Vastus lateralis site is identified by dividing the thigh into thirds, horizontally and vertically. (**C**) Deltoid muscle site is located by palpating lower edge of acromion process.

The medication volume that can be administered intramuscularly varies based on the intended site. Generally, 1 to 4 mL is the accepted volume range, with no more than 1 to 2 mL given at the deltoid site. The less-developed muscles of children and older people limit the intramuscular injection to 1 to 2 mL.

According to the CDC (2012) and current review of evidence (Crawford & Johnson, 2012), aspiration is not required for intramuscular injections. Some literature suggests aspiration *may* be indicated when administering large molecule medications such as penicillin (Crawford & Johnson, 2012). Consult facility policy and manufacturer recommendations to ensure safe administration.

Refer to Box 7-1 in Skill 7 for techniques for reducing discomfort when injecting medications subcutaneously or intramuscularly.

Table 8-2 INTRAMUSCULAR SITE SELECTION

AGE OF PATIENT	RECOMMENDED SITE
Infants	Vastus lateralis
Toddlers (1–2 years)	Vastus lateralis (preferred) or deltoid
Child/Adolescent (3–18 years)	Deltoid (preferred) or vastus lateralis
Adults	Deltoid or ventrogluteal

MEDICATION TYPE	RECOMMENDED SITE
Biologicals (infants and young children)	Vastus lateralis
Biologicals (older children and adults)	Deltoid
Hepatitis B/Rabies	Deltoid
Medications that are known to be irritating, viscous, or oily solutions	Ventrogluteal

(Adapted from Centers for Disease Control and Prevention (CDC). (2012). *The pink book: Appendices. Epidemiology and prevention of vaccine preventable diseases* (11th ed.). Appendix D. Vaccine administration. Vaccine administration guidelines. Available www.cdc.gov/vaccines/pubs/pinkbook/pinkappendx. htm#appd; Centers for Disease Control and Prevention (CDC). (2008). *Needle length and injection site of intramuscular injections.* Available http://www.cdc.gov/vaccines/ed/encounter08/Downloads/Table7.pdf; and Nicoll, L., & Hesby, A. (2002). Intramuscular injection: An integrative research review and guideline for evidence-based practice. *Applied Nursing Research, 16*(2), 149–162.)

Table 8-3 PATIENT POSITIONING

INJECTION SITE	PATIENT POSITION
Deltoid	Patient may sit or stand. A child may be held in an adult's lap.
Ventrogluteal	Patient may stand, sit, lie laterally, and lie supine.
Vastus lateralis	Patient may sit or lie supine. Infants and young children may lie supine or be held in an adult's lap.

(Adapted from Centers for Disease Control and Prevention (CDC). (2012). *The pink book: Appendices. Epidemiology and prevention of vaccine preventable diseases* (11th ed.). Appendix D. Vaccine administration. Vaccine administration guidelines. Available www.cdc.gov/vaccines/pubs/pinkbook/pinkappendx.htm#appd)

DELEGATION CONSIDERATIONS

The administration of an intramuscular injection is not delegated to nursing assistive personnel (NAP) or to unlicensed assistive personnel (UAP). Depending on the state's nurse practice act and the organization's policies and procedures, the administration of an intramuscular injection may be delegated to licensed practical/vocational nurses (LPN/LVNs). The decision to delegate must be based on careful analysis of the patient's needs and circumstances, as well as the qualifications of the person to whom the task is being delegated.

EQUIPMENT

- Gloves
- Additional PPE, as indicated
- Medication
- Sterile syringe and needle of appropriate size and gauge
- Antimicrobial swab
- Small gauze square
- Computer-generated Medication Administration Record (CMAR) or Medication Administration Record (MAR)

ASSESSMENT

Assess the patient for any allergies. Check the expiration date before administering the medication. Assess the appropriateness of the drug for the patient. Verify patient name, dose, route, and time of administration. Review assessment and laboratory data that may influence drug administration. Assess the site on the patient where the injection is to be given. Avoid any site that is bruised, tender, hard, swollen, inflamed, or scarred.

(continued)

SKILL 8 | ADMINISTERING AN INTRAMUSCULAR INJECTION continued

Assess the patient's knowledge of the medication. If the patient has deficient knowledge about the medication, this may be the appropriate time to begin education about it. If the medication may affect the patient's vital signs, assess them before administration. If the medication is intended for pain relief, assess the patient's pain before and after administration.

NURSING DIAGNOSIS

Determine related factors for the nursing diagnoses based on the patient's current status. Appropriate diagnoses may include:

- Acute Pain
- Anxiety
- Risk for Injury

OUTCOME IDENTIFICATION AND PLANNING

The expected outcome to achieve when administering an intramuscular injection is that the patient receives the medication via the intramuscular route. Other outcomes that may be appropriate include the following: the patient's anxiety is decreased; the patient does not experience adverse effects; and the patient understands and complies with the medication regimen.

IMPLEMENTATION

ACTION	RATIONALE
1. Gather equipment. Check each medication order against the original order in the medical record according to facility policy. Clarify any inconsistencies. Check the patient's chart for allergies.	This comparison helps to identify errors that may have occurred when orders were transcribed. The primary care provider's order is the legal record of medication orders for each facility.
2. Know the actions, special nursing considerations, safe dose ranges, purpose of administration, and adverse effects of the medications to be administered. Consider the appropriateness of the medication for this patient.	This knowledge aids the nurse in evaluating the therapeutic effect of the medication in relation to the patient's disorder and can also be used to educate the patient about the medication.
3. Perform hand hygiene.	Hand hygiene prevents the spread of microorganisms.
4. Move the medication cart to the outside of the patient's room or prepare for administration in the medication area.	Organization facilitates error-free administration and saves time.
5. Unlock the medication cart or drawer. Enter pass code and scan employee identification, if required.	Locking the cart or drawer safeguards each patient's medication supply. Hospital accrediting organizations require medication carts to be locked when not in use. Entering pass code and scanning ID allows only authorized users into the system and identifies the user for documentation by the computer.
6. **Prepare medications for one patient at a time.**	This prevents errors in medication administration.
7. Read the CMAR/MAR and select the proper medication from unit stock or the patient's medication drawer.	This is the *first* check of the label.
8. Compare the label with the CMAR/MAR. Check expiration dates and perform calculations, if necessary. Scan the bar code on the package, if required.	This is the *second* check of the label. Verify calculations with another nurse to ensure safety, if necessary.
9. If necessary, withdraw medication from an ampule or vial as described in Skills 3 and 4.	
10. **Depending on facility policy, the third check of the label may occur at this point. If so, when all medications for one patient have been prepared, recheck the labels with the CMAR/MAR before taking the medications to the patient.**	This *third* check ensures accuracy and helps to prevent errors. *Note:* Many facilities require the *third* check to occur at the bedside, after identifying the patient and before administration.

ACTION

11. Lock the medication cart before leaving it.

12. Transport medications to the patient's bedside carefully, and keep the medications in sight at all times.

13. Ensure that the patient receives the medications at the correct time.

14. Perform hand hygiene and put on PPE, if indicated.

15. Identify the patient. Compare the information with the CMAR/MAR. The patient should be identified using at least two methods (The Joint Commission, 2013):

    a. Check the name on the patient's identification band.
    b. Check the identification number on the patient's identification band.
    c. Check the birth date on the patient's identification band.
    d. Ask the patient to state his or her name and birth date, based on facility policy.

16. Close the door to the room or pull the bedside curtain.

17. Complete necessary assessments before administering medications. Check the patient's allergy bracelet or ask the patient about allergies. Explain the purpose and action of the medication to the patient.

18. Scan the patient's bar code on the identification band, if required (Figure 2).

RATIONALE

Locking the cart or drawer safeguards the patient's medication supply. Hospital accrediting organizations require medication carts to be locked when not in use.

Careful handling and close observation prevent accidental or deliberate disarrangement of medications.

Check agency policy, which may allow for administration within a period of 30 minutes before or 30 minutes after the designated time.

Hand hygiene and PPE prevent the spread of microorganisms. PPE is required based on transmission precautions.

Identifying the patient ensures the right patient receives the medications and helps prevent errors. The patient's room number or physical location is not used as an identifier (The Joint Commission, 2013). Replace the identification band if it is missing or inaccurate in any way.

This requires a response from the patient, but illness and strange surroundings often cause patients to be confused.

This provides patient privacy.

Assessment is a prerequisite to administration of medications. Explanation provides rationale, increases knowledge, and reduces anxiety.

Provides an additional check to ensure that the medication is given to the right patient.

FIGURE 2 Scanning bar code on the patient's identification bracelet. *(Photo by B. Proud.)*

(continued)

SKILL 8 ADMINISTERING AN INTRAMUSCULAR INJECTION *continued*

ACTION	RATIONALE
19. Based on facility policy, the third check of the label may occur at this point. If so, recheck the labels with the CMAR/MAR before administering the medications to the patient.	Many facilities require the *third* check to occur at the bedside, after identifying the patient and before administration. If facility policy directs the *third* check at this time, this *third* check ensures accuracy and helps to prevent errors.
20. Put on clean gloves.	Gloves help prevent exposure to contaminants.
21. Select an appropriate administration site.	Selecting the appropriate site prevents injury.
22. Assist the patient to the appropriate position for the site chosen. See Table 8-3. Drape, as needed, to expose only the site area being used.	Appropriate positioning for the site chosen prevents injury. Draping helps maintain the patient's privacy.
23. Identify the appropriate landmarks for the site chosen.	Good visualization is necessary to establish the correct site location and to avoid tissue damage.
24. Cleanse the area around the injection site with an antimicrobial swab. Use a firm, circular motion while moving outward from the injection site. Allow the area to dry.	Pathogens on the skin can be forced into the tissues by the needle. Moving from the center outward prevents contamination of the site. Allowing skin to dry prevents introducing alcohol into the tissue, which can be irritating and uncomfortable.
25. Remove the needle cap by pulling it straight off. Hold the syringe in your dominant hand between the thumb and forefinger.	This technique lessens the risk of an accidental needlestick and also prevents inadvertently unscrewing the needle from the barrel of the syringe.
26. Displace the skin in a Z-track manner. Pull the skin down or to one side about 1 inch (2.5 cm) with your nondominant hand and hold the skin and tissue in this position (Figure 3). (See the accompanying Skill Variation for information on administering an intramuscular injection without using the Z-track technique.)	Z-track technique is recommended for all intramuscular injections to ensure medication does not leak back along the needle track and into the subcutaneous tissue (Nicoll & Hesby, 2002; Zimmerman, 2010). This technique reduces pain and discomfort, particularly for patients receiving injections over an extended period. The Z-track method is also suggested for older patients who have decreased muscle mass. Some agents, such as iron, are best given via the Z-track method due to the irritation and discoloration associated with this agent.

A   B   C   D

FIGURE 3 Z-track or zigzag technique is recommended for intramuscular injections. (**A**) Normal skin and tissues. (**B**) Moving skin to one side. (**C**) Needle is inserted at a 90-degree angle. (**D**) Once needle is withdrawn, displaced tissue is allowed to return to its normal position, preventing solution from escaping from muscle tissue.

ACTION

27. Quickly dart the needle into the tissue so that the needle is perpendicular to the patient's body (Figure 4). This should ensure that the medication is administered using an injection angle between 72 and 90 degrees.

28. As soon as the needle is in place, use the thumb and forefinger of your nondominant hand to hold the lower end of the syringe. Slide your dominant hand to the end of the plunger. Inject the solution slowly (10 sec/mL of medication).

29. Once the medication has been instilled, wait 10 seconds before withdrawing the needle.

30. Withdraw the needle smoothly and steadily at the same angle at which it was inserted, supporting tissue around the injection site with your nondominant hand.

31. Apply gentle pressure at the site with a dry gauze (Figure 5). **Do not massage the site.**

RATIONALE

A quick injection is less painful. Inserting the needle at a 72- to 90-degree angle facilitates entry into muscle tissue.

Moving the syringe could cause damage to the tissues and inadvertent administration into an incorrect area. Rapid injection of the solution creates pressure in the tissues, resulting in discomfort. According to the CDC (2012) and current review of evidence (Crawford & Johnson, 2012), aspiration is not required for intramuscular injections. Some literature suggests aspiration *may* be indicated when administering large molecule medications such as penicillin (Crawford & Johnson, 2012). Consult facility policy and manufacturer recommendations to ensure safe administration.

Allows medication to begin to diffuse into the surrounding muscle tissue (Nicoll & Hesby, 2002).

Slow withdrawal of the needle pulls the tissues and causes discomfort. Applying counter traction around the injection site helps to prevent pulling on the tissue as the needle is withdrawn. Removing the needle at the same angle at which it was inserted minimizes tissue damage and discomfort for the patient.

Light pressure causes less trauma and irritation to the tissues. Massaging can force medication into subcutaneous tissues.

FIGURE 4 Darting needle into tissue.

FIGURE 5 Applying pressure at injection site.

32. Do not recap the used needle. Engage the safety shield or needle guard, if present. Discard the needle and syringe in the appropriate receptacle.

33. Assist the patient to a position of comfort.

 34. Remove gloves and additional PPE, if used. Perform hand hygiene.

Proper disposal of the needle prevents injury.

This provides for the well-being of the patient.

Removing PPE properly reduces the risk for infection transmission and contamination of other items. Hand hygiene prevents the spread of microorganisms.

(continued)

SKILL 8 | ADMINISTERING AN INTRAMUSCULAR INJECTION continued

ACTION	RATIONALE
35. Document the administration of the medication immediately after administration. See Documentation section below.	Timely documentation helps to ensure patient safety.
36. Evaluate the patient's response to the medication within the appropriate time frame. Assess site, if possible, within 2 to 4 hours after administration.	The patient needs to be evaluated for therapeutic and adverse effects from the medication. Visualization of the site allows for assessment of any untoward effects.

EVALUATION

The expected outcomes are met when the patient receives the medication via the intramuscular route; the patient's anxiety is decreased; the patient does not experience adverse effects or injury; and the patient understands and complies with the medication regimen.

DOCUMENTATION

Guidelines

Record each medication given on the CMAR/MAR or record using the required format, including date, time, and the site of administration, immediately after administration. If using a bar-code system, medication administration is automatically recorded when the bar code is scanned. PRN medications require documentation of the reason for administration. Prompt recording avoids the possibility of accidentally repeating the administration of the drug. If the drug was refused or omitted, record this in the appropriate area on the medication record and notify the primary care provider. This verifies the reason medication was omitted and ensures that the primary care provider is aware of the patient's condition.

UNEXPECTED SITUATIONS AND ASSOCIATED INTERVENTIONS

- *You stick yourself with the needle before injection:* Discard needle and syringe appropriately. Follow agency policy regarding needlestick injury. Prepare new syringe with medication and administer to patient. Complete appropriate paperwork and follow facility's policy regarding accidental needlesticks.
- *You stick yourself with the needle after injection:* Discard needle and syringe appropriately. Follow agency policy regarding needlestick injury. Complete appropriate paperwork and follow facility's policy regarding accidental needlesticks.
- *During injection, the patient pulls away from the needle before the medication is delivered fully:* Remove and appropriately discard needle. Attach a new needle to syringe and administer remaining medication at a different site. Document events and interventions, according to facility policy.
- *While injecting the needle into the patient, you hit patient's bone:* Withdraw and discard the needle. Apply a new needle to the syringe and administer in an alternate site. Document incident in patient's medical record. Notify primary care provider. Complete appropriate paperwork related to special events, according to facility policy.

SPECIAL CONSIDERATIONS

General Considerations

- Ongoing assessment is an important part of nursing care for both evaluation of patient response to administered medications and early detection of adverse effects. If an adverse effect is suspected, withhold further medication doses and notify the patient's primary care provider. Additional intervention is based on the type of reaction and patient assessment.

Infant and Child Considerations

- The vastus lateralis is the preferred site for intramuscular injections in infants.

Older Adult Considerations

- Muscle mass atrophies as a person ages. Take care to evaluate the patient's muscle mass and body composition. Use appropriate needle length and gauge for patient's body composition. Choose appropriate site based on the patient's body composition.

Home Care Considerations

- Encourage patients to consult the policies of their local government regarding contaminated and sharps waste disposal. Explain that needles and syringes should be disposed of in a hard, plastic container. Liquid detergent or liquid fabric softener containers are good choices. Glass containers should not be used.
- Reuse of syringes in the home setting is not recommended.

SKILL VARIATION — Administering an Intramuscular Injection Without Using the Z-Track Technique

The Z-track technique is recommended for all intramuscular injections to ensure medication does not leak back along the needle track and into the subcutaneous tissue (Nicoll & Hesby, 2002; Zimmerman, 2010). This technique reduces pain and discomfort, particularly for patients receiving injections over an extended period. The Z-track method is also suggested for older patients who have decreased muscle mass. Some agents, such as iron, are best given via the Z-track method due to the irritation and discoloration associated with this agent. If the nurse chooses not to use the Z-Track technique, the skin should be stretched flat between two fingers and held taut for needle insertion. Prepare medication as outlined in steps 1–13 above (Skill 8). To administer the injection:

1. Perform hand hygiene and put on PPE, as indicated.

2. Identify the patient.

3. Explain the procedure to the patient.
4. Close the door to the room or pull the bedside curtain.
5. Complete necessary assessments before administering medications. Check the patient's allergy bracelet or ask the patient about allergies. Explain the purpose and action of the medication to the patient.
6. Scan the patient's bar code on the identification band, if required.
7. Based on facility policy, the third check of the label may occur at this point. If so, recheck the labels with the CMAR/MAR before administering the medications to the patient.
8. Put on clean gloves.
9. Select an appropriate administration site.

10. Assist the patient to the appropriate position for the site chosen. Drape, as needed, to expose only site area to be used.
11. Identify the appropriate landmarks for the site chosen with your nondominant hand.
12. Clean the area around the injection site with an antimicrobial swab. Use a firm, circular motion while moving outward from the injection site. Allow the area to dry.
13. Remove the needle cap by pulling it straight off. Hold the syringe in your dominant hand between the thumb and forefinger.
14. Stretch the skin flat between two fingers and hold taut for needle insertion.
15. Quickly dart the needle into the tissue so that the needle is perpendicular to the patient's body. This should ensure that it is given using an injection angle between 72 and 90 degrees.
16. As soon as the needle is in place, use your thumb and forefinger of your nondominant hand to hold the lower end of the syringe. Slide your dominant hand to the end of the plunger.
17. Inject the solution slowly (10 sec/mL of medication).
18. Withdraw the needle smoothly and steadily at the same angle at which it was inserted, supporting tissue around the injection site with your nondominant hand.
19. Apply gentle pressure at the site with a dry gauze.
20. Do not recap the used needle. Engage the safety shield or needle guard. Discard the needle and syringe in the appropriate receptacle.
21. Assist the patient to a position of comfort.
22. Remove gloves and additional PPE, if used. Perform hand hygiene.
23. Document administration of the medication on the CMAR/MAR immediately after performing the procedure.
24. Evaluate the patient's response to the medication within the appropriate time frame. Assess site, if possible, within 2 to 4 hours after administration.

EVIDENCE FOR PRACTICE ▶

INTRAMUSCULAR INJECTIONS AND ADMINISTRATION SITE CHOICE

Safe medication administration, including the administration of intramuscular (IM) injections, is an expected competency for nurses. The focus of evidence-based practice and recommendation in the recent nursing literature advocate use of the ventrogluteal site over the dorsogluteal site, to avoid damage to the sciatic nerve. Are nurses incorporating current best practice into their delivery of nursing care?

Related Research

Walsh, L., & Brophy, K. (2010). Staff nurses' sites of choice for administering intramuscular injections to adult patients in the acute care setting. *Journal of Advanced Nursing*, 67(5), 1034–1040.

(continued)

SKILL 8 ADMINISTERING AN INTRAMUSCULAR INJECTION continued

A convenience sample of nurses employed in acute care settings was accessed through a database at a professional association. A questionnaire was sent to 652 nurses; 264 questionnaires were returned, a response rate of 42.2%. Nurses responding to the survey preferentially used the dorsogluteal site over the ventrogluteal site. Only 15.2% of nurses based site selection on recommendations in the nursing literature. Site selection varied significantly with age, level of preparation, years in nursing, and knowledge of nerve injury as a complication with the selected site. The authors concluded nurses are not using the ventrogluteal site for IM injections in adults as recommended in the nursing literature.

Relevance for Nursing Practice
Nurses have a responsibility to provide professional and safe nursing care. This involves maintaining current knowledge and incorporating evidenced-based guidelines and best practices into care provided to patients. Nurses must take responsibility for keeping abreast of current practice guidelines and maintaining involvement in the decision-making process for health care facilities' policies and procedures to ensure safe patient care. In addition, there is a need to explore why nurses are not using current guidelines as recommended in the nursing literature.

SKILL 9 ADMINISTERING A CONTINUOUS SUBCUTANEOUS INFUSION: APPLYING AN INSULIN PUMP

Some medications, such as insulin and morphine, may be administered continuously via the subcutaneous route. Continuous subcutaneous insulin infusion (CSII or insulin pump) allows for multiple preset rates of insulin delivery. This system uses a small, computerized reservoir that delivers insulin via tubing through a small plastic cannula or needle inserted into the subcutaneous tissue. The pump is programmed to deliver multiple preset rates of insulin. The settings can be adjusted for exercise and illness, and bolus dose delivery can be timed in relation to meals. It is recommended that the site is changed every 2 to 3 days to prevent tissue damage or absorption problems (American Association of Diabetes Educators, 2008). Advantages of continuous subcutaneous medication infusion include the longer rate of absorption via the subcutaneous route and convenience for the patient. There are many different manufacturers of insulin pumps. Nurses need to be familiar with the particular pump in use by their patient and to refer to the specific manufacturer's recommendations for use.

DELEGATION CONSIDERATIONS

The administration of a continuous subcutaneous infusion using an insulin pump is not delegated to nursing assistive personnel (NAP) or to unlicensed assistive personnel (UAP). Depending on the state's nurse practice act and the organization's policies and procedures, the management of an insulin pump in some settings may be delegated to licensed practical/vocational nurses (LPN/LVNs) who have received appropriate training. The decision to delegate must be based on careful analysis of the patient's needs and circumstances, as well as the qualifications of the person to whom the task is being delegated.

EQUIPMENT

- Insulin pump
- Pump syringe and vial of insulin or prefilled cartridge, as ordered
- Sterile infusion set
- Insertion (triggering) device
- Needle (24- or 22-gauge, or blunt-ended needle)
- Antimicrobial swabs
- Sterile non-occlusive dressing

- Computer-generated Medication Administration Record (CMAR) or Medication Administration Record (MAR)
- Disposable gloves
- Additional PPE, as indicated

ASSESSMENT

Assess the patient for any allergies. Check the expiration date before administering the medication. Assess the appropriateness of the drug for the patient. Review assessment and laboratory data that may influence drug administration. Verify patient name, dose, route, and time of administration. Assess the infusion site. Typical infusion sites include those areas used for subcutaneous insulin injection. Assess the area where the pump is to be applied. Do not place the pump on skin that is irritated or broken down.

Assess the patient's knowledge of the medication. If the patient has a knowledge deficit about the medication, this may be the appropriate time to begin education about it. Assess the patient's blood glucose level as appropriate or as ordered.

NURSING DIAGNOSIS

Determine related factors for the nursing diagnoses based on the patient's current status. Appropriate nursing diagnoses may include:

- Deficient Knowledge
- Risk for Unstable Blood Glucose Level
- Risk for Infection

OUTCOME IDENTIFICATION AND PLANNING

The expected outcome is that the device is applied successfully and medication is administered correctly. Other outcomes that may be appropriate include the following: the patient understands the rationale for the pump use and mechanism of action; the patient experiences no allergy response; the patient's skin remains intact; pump is applied using aseptic technique; and the patient does not experience unstable blood glucose levels or adverse effect.

IMPLEMENTATION

ACTION	RATIONALE
1. Gather equipment. Check each medication order against the original order in the medical record, according to facility policy. Clarify any inconsistencies. Check the patient's chart for allergies.	This comparison helps to identify errors that may have occurred when orders were transcribed. The primary care provider's order is the legal record of medication orders for each facility.
2. Know the actions, special nursing considerations, safe dose ranges, purpose of administration, and adverse effects of the medications to be administered. Consider the appropriateness of the medication for this patient.	This knowledge aids the nurse in evaluating the therapeutic effect of the medication in relation to the patient's disorder and can also be used to educate the patient about the medication.
3. Perform hand hygiene.	Hand hygiene prevents the spread of microorganisms.
4. Move the medication cart to the outside of the patient's room or prepare for administration in the medication area.	Organization facilitates error-free administration and saves time.
5. Unlock the medication cart or drawer. Enter pass code and scan employee identification, if required.	Locking the cart or drawer safeguards each patient's medication supply. Hospital accrediting organizations require medication carts to be locked when not in use. Entering pass code and scanning ID allows only authorized users into the system and identifies the user for documentation by the computer.
6. Prepare medications for one patient at a time.	This prevents errors in medication administration.
7. Read the CMAR/MAR and select the proper medication from unit stock or the patient's medication drawer.	This is the *first* check of the label.

(continued)

SKILL 9 ADMINISTERING A CONTINUOUS SUBCUTANEOUS INFUSION: APPLYING AN INSULIN PUMP continued

ACTION	RATIONALE
8. Compare the label with the CMAR/MAR. Check expiration dates and perform calculations, if necessary. Scan the bar code on the package, if required.	This is the *second* check of the label. Verify calculations with another nurse to ensure safety, if necessary.
9. Attach a blunt-ended needle or a small-gauge needle to a syringe. Follow Skill 4 to prepare insulin from a vial, if necessary. Prepare enough insulin to last the patient 2 to 3 days, plus 30 units for priming tubing. If using a prepackaged insulin syringe or cartridge, remove from packaging.	Patient will wear pump for up to 3 days without changing syringe or tubing.
10. Depending on facility policy, the third check of the label may occur at this point. If so, when all medications for one patient have been prepared, recheck the labels with the CMAR/MAR before taking the medications to the patient.	This *third* check ensures accuracy and helps to prevent errors. *Note:* Many facilities require the *third* check to occur at the bedside, after identifying the patient and before administration.
11. Lock the medication cart before leaving it.	Locking the cart or drawer safeguards the patient's medication supply. Hospital accrediting organizations require medication carts to be locked when not in use.
12. Transport medications to the patient's bedside carefully, and keep the medications in sight at all times.	Careful handling and close observation prevent accidental or deliberate disarrangement of medications.
13. Ensure that the patient receives the medications at the correct time.	Check agency policy, which may allow for administration within a period of 30 minutes before or 30 minutes after the designated time.
14. Perform hand hygiene and put on PPE, if indicated.	Hand hygiene and PPE prevent the spread of microorganisms. PPE is required based on transmission precautions.
15. Identify the patient. Compare the information with the CMAR/MAR. The patient should be identified using at least two methods (The Joint Commission, 2013):	Identifying the patient ensures the right patient receives the medications and helps prevent errors. The patient's room number or physical location is not used as an identifier (The Joint Commission, 2013). Replace the identification band if it is missing or inaccurate in any way.
a. Check the name on the patient's identification band.	
b. Check the identification number on the patient's identification band.	
c. Check the birth date on the patient's identification band.	
d. Ask the patient to state his or her name and birth date, based on facility policy.	This requires a response from the patient, but illness and strange surroundings often cause patients to be confused.
16. Close the door to the room or pull the bedside curtain.	This provides patient privacy.
17. Complete necessary assessments before administering medications. Check the patient's allergy bracelet or ask the patient about allergies. Explain the purpose and action of the medication to the patient.	Assessment is a prerequisite to administration of medications. Explanation provides rationale, increases knowledge, and reduces anxiety.
18. Scan the patient's bar code on the identification band, if required (Figure 1).	Provides an additional check to ensure that the medication is given to the right patient.
19. Based on facility policy, the third check of the label may occur at this point. If so, recheck the labels with the CMAR/MAR before administering the medications to the patient.	Many facilities require the *third* check to occur at the bedside, after identifying the patient and before administration. If facility policy directs the *third* check at this time, this *third* check ensures accuracy and helps to prevent errors.
20. Perform hand hygiene. Put on gloves.	Hand hygiene prevents the spread of microorganisms. Gloves prevent contact with blood and body fluids.

ACTION

21. Remove the cap from the syringe or insulin cartridge (Figure 2). Attach sterile tubing to the syringe or insulin cartridge. Open the pump and place the syringe or cartridge in compartment according to manufacturer's directions (Figure 3). Close the pump.

FIGURE 1 Scanning bar code on patient's identification bracelet. *(Photo by B. Proud.)*

22. Initiate priming of the tubing, according to manufacturer's directions. Program the pump according to manufacturer's recommendations following primary care provider's orders (Figure 4). **Check for any bubbles in the tubing.**

FIGURE 3 Placing syringe or cartridge in compartment according to manufacturer's directions.

23. Activate the delivery device. Place the needle between prongs of the insertion device with the sharp edge facing out. Push insertion set down until a click is heard.

24. Select an appropriate administration site.

25. Assist the patient to the appropriate position for the site chosen. Drape, as needed, to expose only site area to be used.

RATIONALE

Tubing must be attached correctly and syringe must be placed in pump correctly for insulin delivery.

FIGURE 2 Removing cap from syringe or insulin cartridge.

Removing all the air from the tubing and correct programming of pump ensures the patient receives the correct dose of insulin.

FIGURE 4 Programming pump according to manufacturer's recommendations following primary care provider's orders.

To ensure correct placement of insulin pump needle, an insertion device must be used.

Appropriate site prevents injury.

Appropriate site prevents injury. Draping maintains privacy and warmth.

(continued)

SKILL 9 ADMINISTERING A CONTINUOUS SUBCUTANEOUS INFUSION: APPLYING AN INSULIN PUMP continued

26. Identify the appropriate landmarks for the site chosen.

27. Cleanse area around injection site with antimicrobial swab (Figure 5). Use a firm, circular motion while moving outward from insertion site. Allow antiseptic to dry.

28. Remove paper from adhesive backing. Remove the needle guard. Pinch skin at insertion site, press insertion device on site, and press release button to insert needle. Remove triggering device.

29. Apply sterile occlusive dressing over the insertion site, if not part of the insertion device. Attach the pump to patient's clothing, as desired (Figure 6).

Good visualization is necessary to establish the correct site location and to avoid tissue damage.

Pathogens on the skin can be forced into the tissues by the needle. Moving from the center outward prevents contamination of the site. Allowing skin to dry prevents introducing alcohol into the tissue, which can be irritating and uncomfortable.

To ensure delivery of insulin into subcutaneous tissue, a skin fold is made with a pinch *before* insertion of the medication.

Dressing prevents contamination of site. Pump can be dislodged easily if not attached securely to patient.

FIGURE 5 Cleansing area around injection site with antimicrobial swab.

FIGURE 6 Insulin pump in place.

30. Assist the patient to a position of comfort.

31. Discard the needle and syringe in the appropriate receptacle.

 32. Remove gloves and additional PPE, if used. Perform hand hygiene.

33. Document the administration of the medication immediately after administration. See Documentation section below.

34. Evaluate the patient's response to the medication within the appropriate time frame. Monitor the patient's blood glucose levels, as appropriate, or as ordered.

This provides for the well-being of the patient.

Proper disposal of the needle prevents injury.

Removing PPE properly reduces the risk for infection transmission and contamination of other items. Hand hygiene prevents the spread of microorganisms.

Timely documentation helps to ensure patient safety.

Patient needs to be evaluated to ensure that the pump is delivering the drug appropriately. The patient needs to be evaluated for therapeutic and adverse effects from the medication.

EVALUATION

The expected outcomes are met when the patient receives insulin from the attached pump successfully without hypo- or hyperglycemic effects noted; the patient understands the rationale for the pump attachment; the patient experiences no allergy response; the patient's skin remains intact; the patient remains infection free; and the patient experiences no or minimal pain.

DOCUMENTATION

Guidelines

Document the application of the pump, the type of insulin used, pump settings, insertion site, and any teaching done with the patient on the CMAR/MAR or record using the required format, including date, time, and the site of administration, immediately after administration. If using a bar-code system, medication administration is automatically recorded when the bar code is scanned. PRN medications require documentation of the reason for administration. Prompt recording avoids the possibility of accidentally repeating the administration of the drug. If the drug was refused or omitted, record this in the appropriate area on the medication record and notify the primary care provider. This verifies the reason medication was omitted and ensures that the primary care provider is aware of the patient's condition.

Sample Documentation

> 9/22/15 1000 Insulin pump inserted by patient on left upper quadrant of abdomen with minimal assistance. Pump filled with 300 units (3 mL) of lispro insulin. Rate set at 1 unit per hour. Patient verbalizes desire to apply pump without assistance when site next changed.
>
> —B. Clapp, RN

UNEXPECTED SITUATIONS AND ASSOCIATED INTERVENTIONS

- *After the pump is attached to the patient, a large amount of air is noted in tubing:* Remove the pump from patient. Obtain new sterile tubing with insertion needle. Prime the tubing and reinsert.

SPECIAL CONSIDERATIONS

General Considerations

- *Patient must rotate site more frequently than every 2 to 3 days due to insulin usage:* Check manufacturer's recommendations. Most pumps are initially set in a smaller mode but can be changed for a larger amount of insulin delivery.
- *Patient is refusing to rotate site at least every 3 days:* Inform the patient that absorption of medication decreases after 3 days, which may increase his or her need for insulin. Rotating sites prevents this decrease in absorption from developing. In addition, sit rotation reduces risk of infection at the site.
- *You note that the insertion site is now erythematous:* Remove the stylet, obtain a new pump setup, and insert at a different site at least 1 inch from old site.
- *Occlusive dressing will not stick due to perspiration:* Apply deodorant around insertion site but not over insertion site. Alternately, apply skin barrier around insertion site but not over insertion site.
- Assess infusion site areas routinely for inflammation, allergic reactions, infection, and lipodystrophy.
- Good hygiene and frequent catheter site changes reduce the risk of site complications. Change catheter site every 2 to 3 days.
- Contact dermatitis is sometimes a problem at the catheter site area. The primary care provider may order topical antibiotics, aloe, vitamin E, or corticosteroids to treat a contact dermatitis.
- Insulin self-administered by the patient through the insulin pump should be communicated to the nurse at the time of administration. This allows for accurate documentation of insulin requirements.
- Ongoing assessment is an important part of nursing care for both evaluation of patient response to administered medications and early detection of adverse effects. If an adverse effect is suspected, withhold further medication doses and notify the patient's primary care provider. Additional intervention is based on type of reaction and patient assessment.

Home Care Considerations

- Encourage patients to consult the policies of their local government regarding contaminated and sharps waste disposal. Explain that needles and other sharps should be disposed of in a hard, plastic container. Liquid detergent or liquid fabric softener containers are good choices. Glass containers should not be used.

SKILL 10 ADMINISTERING MEDICATIONS BY INTRAVENOUS BOLUS OR PUSH THROUGH AN INTRAVENOUS INFUSION

A medication can be administered via the **intravenous (IV) route** as an IV bolus or push. This involves a single injection of a concentrated solution directly into an IV line. Drugs given by IV push are used for intermittent dosing or to treat emergencies. The drug is administered very slowly over at least 1 minute. This can be done manually or by using a syringe pump. Confirm exact administration times by consulting a pharmacist or drug reference. Needleless devices prevent needlesticks and provide access to the intravenous line. Either a blunt-ended cannula or a recessed connection port may be used to administer the medication.

DELEGATION CONSIDERATIONS	The administration of medications by intravenous bolus is not delegated to nursing assistive personnel (NAP) or to unlicensed assistive personnel (UAP). Depending on the state's nurse practice act and the organization's policies and procedures, the administration of specified intravenous medications in some settings may be delegated to licensed practical/vocational nurses (LPN/LVNs) who have received appropriate training. The decision to delegate must be based on careful analysis of the patient's needs and circumstances, as well as the qualifications of the person to whom the task is being delegated.
EQUIPMENT	• Antimicrobial swab • Watch with second hand, or stopwatch • Disposable gloves • Additional PPE, as indicated • Prescribed medication • Syringe with a needleless device or 23- to 25-gauge, 1-inch needle (follow facility policy) • Syringe pump, if necessary • Computer-generated Medication Administration Record (CMAR) or Medication Administration Record (MAR)
ASSESSMENT	Assess the patient for any allergies. Check the expiration date before administering the medication. Assess the appropriateness of the drug for the patient. Assess the compatibility of the ordered medication and the IV fluid. Review assessment and laboratory data that may influence drug administration. Verify the patient's name, dose, route, and time of administration. Assess the patient's IV site, noting any swelling, coolness, leakage of fluid from the IV site, or pain. Assess the patient's knowledge of the medication. If the patient has a knowledge deficit about the medication, this may be the appropriate time to begin education about the medication. If the medication may affect the patient's vital signs, assess them before administration. If the medication is for pain relief, assess the patient's pain before and after administration.
NURSING DIAGNOSIS	Determine related factors for the nursing diagnoses based on the patient's current status. Appropriate nursing diagnoses may include: • Risk for Injury • Risk for Allergy Response • Risk for Infection
OUTCOME IDENTIFICATION AND PLANNING	The expected outcome to achieve is that the medication is given safely via the IV route. Other outcomes that may be appropriate include the following: the patient experiences no adverse effects; the patient experiences no allergy response; the patient is knowledgeable about medication being added by bolus IV; the patient remains infection free; and the patient has no, or decreased, anxiety.

IMPLEMENTATION

ACTION	RATIONALE
1. Gather equipment. Check medication order against the original order in the medical record, according to facility policy. Clarify any inconsistencies. Check the patient's chart for allergies. Verify the compatibility of the medication and IV fluid. Check a drug resource to clarify whether the medication needs to be diluted before administration. Check the administration rate.	This comparison helps to identify errors that may have occurred when orders were transcribed. The primary care provider's order is the legal record of medication orders for each facility. Compatibility of medication and solution prevents complications. Delivers the correct dose of medication as prescribed.
2. Know the actions, special nursing considerations, safe dose ranges, purpose of administration, and adverse effects of the medications to be administered. Consider the appropriateness of the medication for this patient.	This knowledge aids the nurse in evaluating the therapeutic effect of the medication in relation to the patient's disorder and can also be used to educate the patient about the medication.
3. Perform hand hygiene.	Hand hygiene prevents the spread of microorganisms.
4. Move the medication cart to the outside of the patient's room or prepare for administration in the medication area.	Organization facilitates error-free administration and saves time.
5. Unlock the medication cart or drawer. Enter pass code and scan employee identification, if required.	Locking the cart or drawer safeguards each patient's medication supply. Hospital accrediting organizations require medication carts to be locked when not in use. Entering pass code and scanning ID allows only authorized users into the system and identifies the user for documentation by the computer.
6. Prepare medication for one patient at a time.	This prevents errors in medication administration.
7. Read the CMAR/MAR and select the proper medication from unit stock or the patient's medication drawer.	This is the *first* check of the label.
8. Compare the label with the CMAR/MAR. Check expiration dates and perform calculations, if necessary. Scan the bar code on the package, if required.	This is the *second* check of the label. Verify calculations with another nurse to ensure safety, if necessary.
9. If necessary, withdraw medication from an ampule or vial as described in Skills 3 and 4.	
10. Depending on facility policy, the third check of the label may occur at this point. If so, when all medications for one patient have been prepared, recheck the labels with the CMAR/MAR before taking the medications to the patient.	This *third* check ensures accuracy and helps to prevent errors. *Note:* Many facilities require the *third* check to occur at the bedside, after identifying the patient and before administration.
11. Lock the medication cart before leaving it.	Locking the cart or drawer safeguards the patient's medication supply. Hospital accrediting organizations require medication carts to be locked when not in use.
12. Transport medications and equipment to the patient's bedside carefully, and keep the medications in sight at all times.	Careful handling and close observation prevent accidental or deliberate disarrangement of medications. Having equipment available saves time and facilitates performance of the task.
13. Ensure that the patient receives the medications at the correct time.	Check agency policy, which may allow for administration within a period of 30 minutes before or 30 minutes after the designated time.
14. Perform hand hygiene and put on PPE, if indicated.	Hand hygiene and PPE prevent the spread of microorganisms. PPE is required based on transmission precautions.

(continued)

SKILL 10 ADMINISTERING MEDICATIONS BY INTRAVENOUS BOLUS OR PUSH THROUGH AN INTRAVENOUS INFUSION continued

ACTION

15. **Identify the patient. Compare the information with the CMAR/MAR. The patient should be identified using at least two methods** (The Joint Commission, 2013):

a. Check the name on the patient's identification band.

b. Check the identification number on the patient's identification band.

c. Check the birth date on the patient's identification band.

d. Ask the patient to state his or her name and birth date, based on facility policy.

16. Close the door to the room or pull the bedside curtain.

17. Complete necessary assessments before administering medications. Check the patient's allergy bracelet or ask the patient about allergies. Explain the purpose and action of the medication to the patient.

18. Scan the patient's bar code on the identification band, if required.

19. **Based on facility policy, the third check of the label may occur at this point. If so, recheck the label with the CMAR/MAR before administering the medications to the patient.**

20. **Assess IV site for presence of inflammation or infiltration.**

21. If IV infusion is being administered via an infusion pump, pause the pump.

22. Put on clean gloves.

23. Select injection port on tubing that is closest to venipuncture site. Clean port with antimicrobial swab.

24. Uncap syringe. Steady port with your nondominant hand while inserting syringe into center of port.

25. Move your nondominant hand to the section of IV tubing just above the injection port. Fold the tubing between your fingers.

26. Pull back slightly on plunger just until blood appears in tubing.

27. **Inject the medication at the recommended rate** (see Special Considerations on page 57) (Figure 1).

RATIONALE

Identifying the patient ensures the right patient receives the medications and helps prevent errors. The patient's room number or physical location is not used as an identifier (The Joint Commission, 2013). Replace the identification band if it is missing or inaccurate in any way.

This requires a response from the patient, but illness and strange surroundings often cause patients to be confused.

This provides patient privacy.

Assessment is a prerequisite to administration of medications. Explanation provides rationale, increases knowledge, and reduces anxiety.

Provides an additional check to ensure that the medication is given to the right patient.

Many facilities require the *third* check to occur at the bedside, after identifying the patient and before administration. If facility policy directs the *third* check at this time, this *third* check ensures accuracy and helps to prevent errors.

IV medication must be given directly into a vein for safe administration.

Pausing prevents infusion of fluid during bolus administration and activation of pump occlusion alarms.

Gloves prevent contact with blood and body fluids.

Using port closest to the needle insertion site minimizes dilution of medication. Cleaning deters entry of microorganisms when port is punctured.

This supports the injection port and lessens the risk for accidentally dislodging the IV or entering the port incorrectly.

This temporarily stops flow of gravity IV infusion and prevents medication from backing up tubing.

This ensures injection of medication into the bloodstream.

This delivers the correct amount of medication at the proper interval according to manufacturer's directions.

FIGURE 1 Injecting medication while interrupting IV flow. *(Photo by B. Proud.)*

ACTION	RATIONALE
28. Release the tubing. Remove the syringe. Do not recap the used needle, if used. Engage the safety shield or needle guard, if present. Release the tubing and allow the IV fluid to flow. Discard the needle and syringe in the appropriate receptacle.	Proper disposal of the needle prevents injury.
29. Check IV fluid infusion rate. Restart infusion pump, if appropriate.	Injection of bolus may alter fluid infusion rate, if infusing by gravity.
30. Remove gloves and additional PPE, if used. Perform hand hygiene.	Removing PPE properly reduces the risk for infection transmission and contamination of other items. Hand hygiene prevents the spread of microorganisms.
31. Document the administration of the medication immediately after administration. See Documentation section below.	Timely documentation helps to ensure patient safety.
32. Evaluate the patient's response to the medication within the appropriate time frame.	The patient needs to be evaluated for therapeutic and adverse effects from the medication.

EVALUATION

The expected outcomes are met when the medication is safely administered via IV bolus; the patient's anxiety is decreased; the patient does not experience adverse effects; and the patient understands and complies with the medication regimen.

DOCUMENTATION

Guidelines

Document the administration of the medication immediately after administration, including date, time, dose, route of administration, site of administration, and rate of administration on the CMAR/MAR or record using the required format. If using a bar-code system, medication administration is automatically recorded when the bar code is scanned. PRN medications require documentation of the reason for administration. Prompt recording avoids the possibility of accidentally repeating the administration of the drug. If the drug was refused or omitted, record this in the appropriate area on the medication record and notify the primary care provider. This verifies the reason medication was omitted and ensures that the primary care provider is aware of the patient's condition.

UNEXPECTED SITUATIONS AND ASSOCIATED INTERVENTIONS

- *Upon assessing the IV site before administering medication, no blood return is aspirated:* If IV appears patent, without signs of infiltration, and IV fluid infuses without difficulty, proceed with administration. Observe closely for signs and symptoms of infiltration during and after administration.
- *Upon assessing the patient's IV site before administering medication, you note that IV has infiltrated:* Stop IV fluid and remove IV from extremity. Restart IV in a different location. Continue to monitor new IV site as medication is administered.
- *While administering medication, you note a cloudy, white substance forming in the IV tubing:* Stop the IV from flowing and stop administering medication. Clamp IV at the site nearest to the patient. Change administration tubing and restart infusion. Check literature or consult pharmacist regarding compatibility of medication and IV fluid.
- *While you are administering the medication, the patient begins to complain of pain at the IV site:* Stop medication. Assess IV site for any signs of infiltration or phlebitis. Flush the IV with normal saline to check for patency. If the IV site appears within normal limits, resume medication administration at a slower rate.

SPECIAL CONSIDERATIONS

- Facility policy may recommend the following variations when injecting a bolus IV medication:
  - Release folded tubing after each increment of the drug has been administered at the prescribed rate to facilitate delivery of medication.
  - Use a syringe with 1 mL normal saline to flush tubing after an IV bolus is delivered to ensure that residual medication in tubing is not delivered too rapidly. *(continued)*

SKILL 10 ADMINISTERING MEDICATIONS BY INTRAVENOUS BOLUS OR PUSH THROUGH AN INTRAVENOUS INFUSION continued

- Consider how fast IV fluid is flowing to determine whether a flush of normal saline is in order after administering the medication. If IV fluid is flowing less than 50 mL per hour, it may take up to 30 minutes for the medication to reach the patient. This depends on what type of tubing is being used in the agency.
- If the IV is a small gauge (22- to 24-gauge) placed in a small vein, a blood return may not occur even if IV is intact. Also, the patient may complain of stinging and pain at the site while medication is being administered due to irritation of vein. Placing a warm pack over the vein or slowing the rate may relieve discomfort.
- If the medication and IV solution are incompatible, a bolus may be given by flushing the tubing with normal saline before and after the medication bolus. Consult facility policy.
- Ongoing assessment is an important part of nursing care for both evaluation of patient response to administered medications and early detection of adverse effects. If an adverse effect is suspected, withhold further medication doses and notify the patient's primary care provider. Additional intervention is based on type of reaction and patient assessment.

SKILL 11 ADMINISTERING A PIGGYBACK INTERMITTENT INTRAVENOUS INFUSION OF MEDICATION

With intermittent IV infusion, the drug is mixed with a small amount of the IV solution, such as 50 to 100 mL, and administered over a short period at the prescribed interval (e.g., every 4 hours). The administration is most often performed using an IV infusion pump, which requires the nurse to program the infusion rate into the pump. "Smart (computerized) pumps" are being used by many facilities for IV infusions, including intermittent infusions. Smart pumps also require programming of infusion rates by the nurse, but also are able to identify dosing limits and practice guidelines to aid in safe administration. Administration may also be achieved by gravity infusion, which requires the nurse to calculate the infusion rate in drops per minute. The best practice, however, is to use an IV infusion pump.

The IV piggyback delivery system requires the intermittent or additive solution to be placed higher than the primary solution container. An extension hook provided by the manufacturer provides for easy lowering of the main IV container. The port on the primary IV line has a back-check valve that automatically stops the flow of the primary solution, allowing the secondary or piggyback solution to flow when connected. Because manufacturers' designs vary, it is important to check the directions carefully for the systems used in the facility. The nurse is responsible for calculating and regulating the infusion with an infusion pump or manually adjusting the flow rate of the IV intermittent infusion. Needleless devices (recommended by the CDC and the Occupational Safety and Health Administration [OSHA]) prevent needlesticks and provide access to the primary venous line. Either a blunt-ended cannula or a recessed connection port may be used to connect intermittent IV infusions.

DELEGATION CONSIDERATIONS

The administration of medications by intermittent IV infusion is not delegated to nursing assistive personnel (NAP) or to unlicensed assistive personnel (UAP). Depending on the state's nurse practice act and the organization's policies and procedures, the administration of specified IV medications in some settings may be delegated to licensed practical/vocational nurses (LPN/LVNs) who have received appropriate training. The decision to delegate must be based on careful analysis of the patient's needs and circumstances, as well as the qualifications of the person to whom the task is being delegated.

EQUIPMENT

- Medication prepared in labeled small-volume bag
- Short secondary infusion tubing (microdrip or macrodrip)
- IV pump
- Needleless connector, if required, based on facility system
- Antimicrobial swab

- Metal or plastic hook
- IV pole
- Date label for tubing
- Computer-generated Medication Administration Record (CMAR) or Medication Administration Record (MAR)
- PPE, as indicated

ASSESSMENT

Assess the patient for any allergies. Check the expiration date before administering the medication. Assess the appropriateness of the drug for the patient. Assess the compatibility of the ordered medication, diluent, and the infusing IV fluid. Review assessment and laboratory data that may influence drug administration. Verify patient name, dose, route, and time of administration. Assess the patient's knowledge of the medication. If the patient has a knowledge deficit about the medication, this may be the appropriate time to begin education about the medication. If the medication may affect the patient's vital signs, assess them before administration. Assess the IV insertion site, noting any swelling, coolness, leakage of fluid at site, redness, or pain.

NURSING DIAGNOSIS

Determine related factors for the nursing diagnoses based on the patient's current status. Appropriate nursing diagnoses include:

- Risk for Allergy Response
- Risk for Infection

- Risk for Injury

OUTCOME IDENTIFICATION AND PLANNING

The expected outcome to achieve is that the medication is delivered via the intravenous route using sterile technique. Other outcomes that may be appropriate include the following: medication is delivered to the patient in a safe manner and at the appropriate infusion rate; the patient experiences no allergy response; the patient remains infection free; and the patient understands and complies with the medication regimen.

IMPLEMENTATION

ACTION	RATIONALE
1. Gather equipment. Check each medication order against the original order in the medical record, according to facility policy. Clarify any inconsistencies. Check the patient's chart for allergies.	This comparison helps to identify errors that may have occurred when orders were transcribed. The primary care provider order is the legal record of medication orders for each facility.
2. Know the actions, special nursing considerations, safe dose ranges, purpose of administration, and adverse effects of the medications to be administered. Consider the appropriateness of the medication for this patient.	This knowledge aids the nurse in evaluating the therapeutic effect of the medication in relation to the patient's disorder and can also be used to educate the patient about the medication.
3. Perform hand hygiene.	Hand hygiene prevents the spread of microorganisms.
4. Move the medication cart to the outside of the patient's room or prepare for administration in the medication area.	Organization facilitates error-free administration and saves time.
5. Unlock the medication cart or drawer. Enter pass code and scan employee identification, if required.	Locking the cart or drawer safeguards each patient's medication supply. Hospital accrediting organizations require medication carts to be locked when not in use. Entering pass code and scanning ID allows only authorized users into the system and identifies the user for documentation by the computer.
6. Prepare medications for one patient at a time.	This prevents errors in medication administration.
7. Read the CMAR/MAR and select the proper medication from unit stock or the patient's medication drawer.	This is the *first* check of the label.

(continued)

SKILL 11 ADMINISTERING A PIGGYBACK INTERMITTENT INTRAVENOUS INFUSION OF MEDICATION continued

ACTION	RATIONALE
8. Compare the label with the CMAR/MAR. Check expiration dates. Confirm the prescribed or appropriate infusion rate. Calculate the drip rate if using a gravity system. Scan the bar code on the package, if required.	This is the *second* check of the label. Verify calculations with another nurse to ensure safety, if necessary. Infusing medication at an appropriate rate prevents injury.
9. Depending on facility policy, the third check of the label may occur at this point. If so, when all medications for one patient have been prepared, recheck the labels with the CMAR/MAR before taking the medications to the patient.	This *third* check ensures accuracy and helps to prevent errors. *Note:* Many facilities require the *third* check to occur at the bedside, after identifying the patient and before administration.
10. Lock the medication cart before leaving it.	Locking the cart or drawer safeguards the patient's medication supply. Hospital accrediting organizations require medication carts to be locked when not in use.
11. Transport medications to the patient's bedside carefully, and keep the medications in sight at all times.	Careful handling and close observation prevent accidental or deliberate disarrangement of medications.
12. Ensure that the patient receives the medications at the correct time.	Check facility policy, which may allow for administration within a period of 30 minutes before or 30 minutes after the designated time.
13. Perform hand hygiene and put on PPE, if indicated.	Hand hygiene and PPE prevent the spread of microorganisms. PPE is required based on transmission precautions.
14. Identify the patient. Compare the information with the CMAR/MAR. The patient should be identified using at least two methods (The Joint Commission, 2013):	Identifying the patient ensures the right patient receives the medications and helps prevent errors. The patient's room number or physical location is not used as an identifier (The Joint Commission, 2013). Replace the identification band if it is missing or inaccurate in any way.
a. Check the name on the patient's identification band.	
b. Check the identification number on the patient's identification band.	
c. Check the birth date on the patient's identification band.	
d. Ask the patient to state his or her name and birth date, based on facility policy.	This requires a response from the patient, but illness and strange surroundings often cause patients to be confused.
15. Close the door to the room or pull the bedside curtain.	This provides patient privacy.
16. Complete necessary assessments before administering medications. Check the patient's allergy bracelet or ask the patient about allergies. Explain the purpose and action of the medication to the patient.	Assessment is a prerequisite to administration of medications. Explanation provides rationale, increases knowledge, and reduces anxiety.
17. Scan the patient's bar code on the identification band, if required.	Scanning provides an additional check to ensure that the medication is given to the right patient.
18. Based on facility policy, the third check of the label may occur at this point. If so, recheck the labels with the CMAR/MAR before administering the medications to the patient.	Many facilities require the *third* check to occur at the bedside, after identifying the patient and before administration. If facility policy directs the *third* check at this time, this *third* check ensures accuracy and helps to prevent errors.
19. Assess the IV site for the presence of inflammation or infiltration.	IV medication must be given directly into a vein for safe administration.
20. Close the clamp on the short secondary infusion tubing. Using aseptic technique, remove the cap on the tubing spike and the cap on the port of the medication container, taking care to avoid contaminating either end.	Closing the clamp prevents fluid from entering the system until the nurse is ready. Maintaining sterility of the tubing and the medication port prevents contamination.

ACTION	RATIONALE
21. Attach infusion tubing to the medication container by inserting the tubing spike into the port with a firm push and twisting motion, taking care to avoid contaminating either end.	Maintaining sterility of tubing and medication port prevents contamination.
22. Hang piggyback container on IV pole, positioning it higher than primary IV according to manufacturer's recommendations (Figure 1). Use metal or plastic hook to lower primary IV fluid container. (See the accompanying Skill Variation for information on administering an intermittent IV medication using a tandem piggyback setup.)	Position of containers influences the flow of IV fluid into the primary setup.
23. Place label on tubing with appropriate date.	Tubing for piggyback setup may be used for 48 to 96 hours, depending on agency policy. Label allows for tracking of the next date to change the medication.
24. Squeeze drip chamber on tubing and release. Fill to the line or about half full. Open clamp and prime tubing. Close clamp. Place needleless connector on the end of the tubing, using sterile technique, if required.	This removes air from tubing and preserves the sterility of the setup.
25. Use an antimicrobial swab to clean the access port or stopcock above the roller clamp on the primary IV infusion tubing (Figure 2).	This deters entry of microorganisms when the piggyback setup is connected to the port. Backflow valve in the primary line secondary port stops flow of primary infusion while piggyback solution is infusing. Once completed, backflow valves open and flow of primary solution resumes.
26. Connect piggyback setup to the access port or stopcock (Figure 3). If using, turn the stopcock to the open position.	Needleless systems and stopcock setup eliminate the need for a needle and are recommended by the CDC.

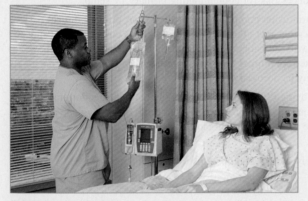

FIGURE 1 Positioning piggyback container on IV pole. *(Photo by B. Proud.)*

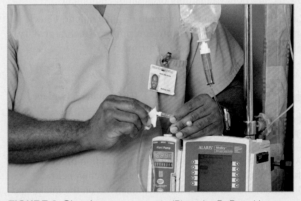

FIGURE 2 Cleaning access port. *(Photo by B. Proud.)*

FIGURE 3 Connecting piggyback setup to access port. *(Photo by B. Proud.)*

(continued)

SKILL 11   ADMINISTERING A PIGGYBACK INTERMITTENT INTRAVENOUS INFUSION OF MEDICATION   continued

ACTION	RATIONALE
27. Open clamp on the secondary tubing. Set rate for secondary infusion on infusion pump and begin infusion (Figure 4). If using gravity infusion, use the roller clamp on the primary infusion tubing to regulate the flow at the prescribed delivery rate (Figure 5). Monitor medication infusion at periodic intervals.	Backflow valve in the primary line secondary port stops flow of primary infusion while piggyback solution is infusing. Once completed, backflow valves open and flow of primary solution resumes. It is important to verify the safe administration rate for each drug to prevent adverse effects.

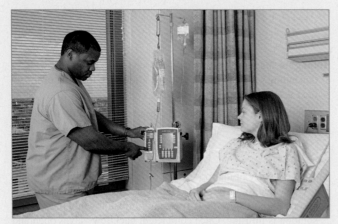

FIGURE 4 Setting rate on infusion pump. *(Photo by B. Proud.)*

FIGURE 5 Using roller clamp on primary infusion tubing to regulate gravity flow. *(Photo by B. Proud.)*

28. Clamp tubing on piggyback set when solution is infused. Follow facility policy regarding disposal of equipment.	Most facilities allow the reuse of tubing for 48 to 96 hours. This reduces risk for contaminating primary IV setup.
29. Raise primary IV fluid container to original height. **Check primary infusion rate on infusion pump. If using gravity infusion, readjust flow rate of primary IV.**	Most infusion pumps automatically restart primary infusion at previous rate after secondary infusion is completed. If using gravity infusion, piggyback medication administration may interrupt normal flow rate of primary IV. Rate readjustment may be necessary.
30. Remove PPE, if used. Perform hand hygiene.	Removing PPE properly reduces the risk for infection transmission and contamination of other items. Hand hygiene prevents the spread of microorganisms.
31. Document the administration of the medication immediately after administration. See Documentation section below. Document the volume of fluid administered on the intake and output record, if necessary.	Timely documentation helps to ensure patient safety.
32. Evaluate the patient's response to the medication within an appropriate time frame. Monitor IV site at periodic intervals.	The patient needs to be evaluated for therapeutic and adverse effects from the medication.

EVALUATION

The expected outcomes are met when the medication is delivered via the IV route using sterile technique; the medication is delivered to the patient in a safe manner and at the appropriate infusion rate; the patient experiences no allergy response; the patient remains infection free; and the patient understands and complies with the medication regimen.

DOCUMENTATION

Guidelines

Document the administration of the medication immediately after administration, including date, time, dose, route of administration, site of administration, and rate of administration on the CMAR/MAR or record using the required format. If using a bar-code system, medication administration is automatically recorded when the bar code is scanned. PRN medications require documentation of the reason for administration. Prompt recording avoids the possibility of accidentally repeating the administration of the drug. If the drug was refused or omitted, record this in the appropriate area on the medication record and notify the primary care provider. This verifies the reason medication was omitted and ensures that the primary care provider is aware of the patient's condition. Document the volume of fluid administered on the intake and output record, if necessary.

UNEXPECTED SITUATIONS AND ASSOCIATED INTERVENTIONS

- *Upon assessing the IV site before administering medication, you note that the IV has infiltrated:* Stop IV fluid and remove the IV from the extremity. Restart the IV in a different location. Continue to monitor the new IV site as medication is administered.
- *While administering medication, you note a cloudy, white substance forming in the IV tubing:* Stop the IV from flowing and stop administering the medication to prevent precipitate from entering the patient's circulation. Clamp the IV at the site nearest to the patient. Replace tubing on primary and secondary infusions. Check the literature regarding incompatibilities of medications before administering. Medication infusion may require a second IV site or flushing of tubing before and after administration, using the tandem system.
- *While you are administering medication, the patient begins to complain of pain at the IV site:* Stop the medication. Assess the IV site for any signs of infiltration or phlebitis. Flush the IV with normal saline to check for patency. If the IV site appears within normal limits, resume medication administration at a slower rate.

SPECIAL CONSIDERATIONS
General Considerations

- An alternate way to prime the secondary tubing, particularly if administration set is in place from a previous infusion, is to "backfill" the secondary tubing. Attach the medication bag to the secondary infusion tubing. Lower the medication bag below the main IV solution container and open the clamp on the secondary infusion tubing. This allows the primary IV solution to flow up the secondary tubing to the drip chamber, "backfilling" the tubing. Allow the solution to enter the drip chamber until the drip chamber is half full. Close the clamp on the secondary tubing and hang the medication container on the IV pole. Proceed with administration by lowering the primary IV container, as described above. This "backfill" method keeps the infusion system intact, preventing both introduction of microorganisms and loss of medication when the tubing is primed. Check facility policy regarding the use of "backfilling."
- Ongoing assessment is an important part of nursing care for both evaluation of patient response to administered medications and early detection of adverse effects. If an adverse effect is suspected, withhold further medication doses and notify the patient's primary care provider. Additional intervention is based on type of reaction and patient assessment.

Infant and Child Considerations

- Infants and small children with fluid restrictions may not tolerate the added IV fluid needed for administration with piggyback or volume-control systems. For these children, consider using the mini-infusion pump (see Skill 12).

SKILL VARIATION   Tandem Piggyback Setup

A tandem delivery setup allows for simultaneous infusion of the primary and secondary IV solutions. Both solution containers are hung at the same height. Tubing for the secondary infusion is attached to an access port below the roller clamp on the primary tubing. There is no back-check valve at the secondary port on the primary line. This type of setup is used infrequently because the solution from the primary IV line will back up into the tandem line if this intermittent infusion is not clamped immediately after it is infused. It requires a second IV infusion pump to control the rate of the secondary infusion (or the use of primary tubing, if using gravity infusion).

Prepare medication as outlined in steps 1–12 above (Skill 11).

1. Perform hand hygiene and put on PPE, if indicated.

2. Identify the patient. The patient should be identified using two methods.

3. Close the door to the room or pull the bedside curtain.

(continued)

SKILL 11 ADMINISTERING A PIGGYBACK INTERMITTENT INTRAVENOUS INFUSION OF MEDICATION continued

SKILL VARIATION Tandem Piggyback Setup continued

4. Complete necessary assessments before administering medications. Check the patient's allergy bracelet or ask the patient about allergies. Explain the purpose and action of the medication to the patient.
5. Scan the patient's bar code on the identification band, if required.
6. Based on facility policy, the third check of the label may occur at this point. If so, recheck the labels with the CMAR/MAR before administering the medications to the patient.
7. Assess the IV site for the presence of inflammation or infiltration.
8. Close the clamp on the secondary infusion tubing. Using aseptic technique, remove the cap on the tubing spike and the cap on the port of the medication container, taking care not to contaminate either end.
9. Attach infusion tubing to the medication container by inserting the tubing spike into the port with a firm push and twisting motion, taking care not to contaminate either end.
10. Hang the secondary container on the IV pole, positioning it at the same height as the primary IV.
11. Place label on tubing with appropriate date.
12. Squeeze drip chamber and release. Fill to the line or about half full. Open clamp and prime tubing. Close clamp. Place needleless connector on the end of the tubing using sterile

technique, if required. Insert tubing into infusion pump, according to manufacturer's directions.
13. Use an antimicrobial swab to clean the access port or stopcock below the roller clamp on the primary IV infusion tubing, usually the port closest to the IV insertion site.
14. Connect the secondary setup to the access port or stopcock. If using, turn the stopcock to the open position.
15. Open the clamp on the secondary tubing. Set rate for secondary infusion on infusion pump. If using gravity infusion, use the roller clamp on the primary infusion tubing to regulate the flow at the prescribed delivery rate. Monitor medication infusion at periodic intervals.
16. Turn off secondary infusion pump. Clamp tubing on secondary set when solution is infused. Remove secondary tubing from access port and cap, or replace connector with a new, capped one, if reusing. Follow facility policy regarding disposal of equipment.
17. Check primary infusion rate.
 18. Remove PPE, if used. Perform hand hygiene.
19. Evaluate the patient's response to the medication within an appropriate time frame. Monitor the IV site at periodic intervals.

SKILL 12 ADMINISTERING AN INTERMITTENT INTRAVENOUS INFUSION OF MEDICATION VIA A MINI-INFUSION PUMP

With intermittent IV infusion, the drug is mixed with a small amount of the IV solution, and administered over a short period at the prescribed interval (e.g., every 4 hours). The mini-infusion pump (syringe pump) for intermittent infusion is battery or electrical operated and allows medication mixed in a syringe to be connected to the primary line and delivered by mechanical pressure applied to the syringe plunger. "Smart (computerized) pumps" are being used by many facilities for IV infusions, including intermittent infusions. Smart pumps also require programming of infusion rates by the nurse, but also are able to identify dosing limits and practice guidelines to aid in safe administration. Needleless devices (recommended by the CDC and the Occupational Safety and Health Administration [OSHA]) prevent needlesticks and provide access to the primary venous line. Either a blunt-ended cannula or a recessed connection port may be used to connect intermittent IV infusions.

DELEGATION CONSIDERATIONS

The administration of medications by intermittent IV infusion is not delegated to nursing assistive personnel (NAP) or to unlicensed assistive personnel (UAP). Depending on the state's nurse practice act and the organization's policies and procedures, the administration of specified IV medications in some settings may be delegated to licensed practical/vocational nurses (LPN/LVNs) who have received appropriate training. The decision to delegate must be based on careful analysis of the patient's needs and circumstances, as well as the qualifications of the person to whom the task is being delegated.

EQUIPMENT	
	• Medication prepared in labeled syringe
	• Mini-infusion pump and tubing
	• Needleless connector, if required, based on facility system
	• Antimicrobial swab
	• Date label for tubing
	• Computer-generated Medication Administration Record (CMAR) or Medication Administration Record (MAR)
	• PPE, as indicated

ASSESSMENT

Assess the patient for any allergies. Check the expiration date before administering medication. Assess the appropriateness of the drug for the patient. Assess the compatibility of the ordered medication, diluent, and the infusing IV fluid. Review assessment and laboratory data that may influence drug administration. Verify patient name, dose, route, and time of administration. Assess the patient's knowledge of the medication. If the patient has a knowledge deficit about the medication, this may be the appropriate time to begin education about the medication. If the medication may affect the patient's vital signs, assess them before administration. Assess the IV insertion site, noting any swelling, coolness, leakage of fluid at site, redness, or pain.

NURSING DIAGNOSIS

Determine related factors for the nursing diagnoses based on the patient's current status. Appropriate nursing diagnoses include:

• Risk for Allergy Response   • Risk for Infection
• Risk for Injury

OUTCOME IDENTIFICATION AND PLANNING

The expected outcome is that the medication is delivered via the IV route using sterile technique. Other outcomes that may be appropriate include the following: medication is delivered to the patient in a safe manner and at the appropriate infusion rate; the patient experiences no allergy response; the patient remains infection free; and the patient understands and complies with the medication regimen.

IMPLEMENTATION

ACTION	RATIONALE
1. Gather equipment. Check each medication order against the original order in the medical record according to facility policy. Clarify any inconsistencies. Check the patient's chart for allergies.	This comparison helps to identify errors that may have occurred when orders were transcribed. The primary care provider's order is the legal record of medication orders for each facility. Compatibility of medication and solution prevents complications.
2. Know the actions, special nursing considerations, safe dose ranges, purpose of administration, and adverse effects of the medications to be administered. Consider the appropriateness of the medication for this patient.	This knowledge aids the nurse in evaluating the therapeutic effect of the medication in relation to the patient's disorder and can also be used to educate the patient about the medication.
3. Perform hand hygiene.	Hand hygiene prevents the spread of microorganisms.
4. Move the medication cart to the outside of the patient's room or prepare for administration in the medication area.	Organization facilitates error-free administration and saves time.
5. Unlock the medication cart or drawer. Enter pass code and scan employee identification, if required.	Locking the cart or drawer safeguards each patient's medication supply. Hospital accrediting organizations require medication carts to be locked when not in use. Entering pass code and scanning ID allows only authorized users into the system and identifies the user for documentation by the computer.

(continued)

SKILL 12 ADMINISTERING AN INTERMITTENT INTRAVENOUS INFUSION OF MEDICATION VIA A MINI-INFUSION PUMP continued

ACTION	RATIONALE
6. Prepare medications for one patient at a time.	This prevents errors in medication administration.
7. Read the CMAR/MAR and select the proper medication from unit stock or the patient's medication drawer.	This is the *first* check of the label.
8. Compare the label with the CMAR/MAR. Check expiration dates. Confirm the prescribed or appropriate infusion rate. Scan the bar code on the package, if required.	This is the *second* check of the label. Verify calculations with another nurse to ensure safety, if necessary. Infusing medication at appropriate rate prevents injury.
9. Depending on facility policy, the third check of the label may occur at this point. If so, when all medications for one patient have been prepared, recheck the labels with the CMAR/MAR before taking the medications to the patient.	This *third* check ensures accuracy and helps to prevent errors. *Note:* Many facilities require the *third* check to occur at the bedside, after identifying the patient and before administration.
10. Lock the medication cart before leaving it.	Locking the cart or drawer safeguards the patient's medication supply. Hospital accrediting organizations require medication carts to be locked when not in use.
11. Transport medications to the patient's bedside carefully, and keep the medications in sight at all times.	Careful handling and close observation prevent accidental or deliberate disarrangement of medications.
12. Ensure that the patient receives the medications at the correct time.	Check agency policy, which may allow for administration within a period of 30 minutes before or 30 minutes after the designated time.
13. Perform hand hygiene and put on PPE, if indicated.	Hand hygiene and PPE prevent the spread of microorganisms. PPE is required based on transmission precautions.
14. Identify the patient. Compare the information with the CMAR/MAR. The patient should be identified using at least two methods (The Joint Commission, 2013):	Identifying the patient ensures the right patient receives the medications and helps prevent errors. The patient's room number or physical location is not used as an identifier (The Joint Commission, 2013). Replace the identification band if it is missing or inaccurate in any way.
a. Check the name on the patient's identification band.	
b. Check the identification number on the patient's identification band.	
c. Check the birth date on the patient's identification band.	
d. Ask the patient to state his or her name and birth date, based on facility policy.	This requires a response from the patient, but illness and strange surroundings often cause patients to be confused.
15. Close the door to the room or pull the bedside curtain.	Provides patient privacy.
16. Complete necessary assessments before administering medications. Check the patient's allergy bracelet or ask the patient about allergies. Explain the purpose and action of the medication to the patient.	Assessment is a prerequisite to administration of medications. Explanation provides rationale, increases knowledge, and reduces anxiety.
17. Scan the patient's bar code on the identification band, if required.	Provides an additional check to ensure that the medication is given to the right patient.
18. Based on facility policy, the third check of the label may occur at this point. If so, recheck the labels with the CMAR/MAR before administering the medications to the patient.	Many facilities require the *third* check to occur at the bedside, after identifying the patient and before administration. If facility policy directs the *third* check at this time, this *third* check ensures accuracy and helps to prevent errors.
19. Assess the IV site for the presence of inflammation or infiltration.	IV medication must be given directly into a vein for safe administration.
20. Using aseptic technique, remove the cap on the tubing and the cap on the syringe, taking care not to contaminate either end.	Maintaining sterility of tubing and medication port prevents contamination.

ACTION	RATIONALE
21. Attach infusion tubing to the syringe, taking care not to contaminate either end.	Maintaining sterility of tubing and medication port prevents contamination.
22. Place label on tubing with appropriate date.	Tubing for piggyback setup may be used for 48 to 96 hours, depending on facility policy. Label allows for tracking of the next date to change.
23. Fill tubing with medication by applying gentle pressure to syringe plunger. Place needleless connector on the end of the tubing, using sterile technique, if required.	This removes air from tubing and maintains sterility.
24. Insert syringe into mini-infusion pump according to manufacturer's directions (Figure 1).	Syringe must fit securely in pump apparatus for proper operation.
25. Use antimicrobial swab to clean the access port or stopcock below the roller clamp on the primary IV infusion tubing, usually the port closest to the IV insertion site (Figure 2).	This deters entry of microorganisms when the piggyback setup is connected to the port. Proper connection allows IV medication to flow into the primary line.
26. Connect the secondary infusion to the primary infusion at the cleansed port (Figure 3).	Allows for delivery of medication.
27. Program the pump to the appropriate rate and begin infusion (Figure 4). Set the alarm if recommended by the manufacturer.	Pump delivers medication at a controlled rate. Alarm is recommended for use with IV lock apparatus.

FIGURE 1 Inserting syringe into mini-infusion pump.

FIGURE 2 Cleaning access port closest to IV insertion site.

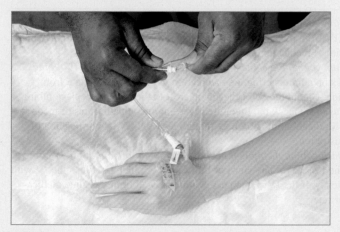

FIGURE 3 Connecting secondary infusion tubing to primary infusion.

FIGURE 4 Programming mini-infusion pump.

(*continued*)

SKILL 12 ADMINISTERING AN INTERMITTENT INTRAVENOUS INFUSION OF MEDICATION VIA A MINI-INFUSION PUMP continued

ACTION	RATIONALE
28. Clamp tubing on secondary set when solution is infused. Remove secondary tubing from access port and cap, or replace connector with a new, capped one, if reusing. Follow facility policy regarding disposal of equipment.	Many facilities allow reuse of tubing for 48 to 96 hours. Replacing connector or needle with a new, capped one maintains system sterility.
29. Check rate of primary infusion.	Administration of secondary infusion may interfere with primary infusion rate.
30. Remove PPE, if used. Perform hand hygiene.	Removing PPE properly reduces the risk for infection transmission and contamination of other items. Hand hygiene prevents the spread of microorganisms.
31. Document the administration of the medication immediately after administration. See Documentation section below. Document the volume of fluid administered on the intake and output record, if necessary.	Timely documentation helps to ensure patient safety.
32. Evaluate the patient's response to the medication within appropriate time frame. Monitor IV site at periodic intervals.	The patient needs to be evaluated for therapeutic and adverse effects from the medication.

EVALUATION

The expected outcomes are met when the medication is delivered via the IV route using sterile technique; the medication is delivered to the patient in a safe manner and at the appropriate infusion rate; the patient experiences no allergy response; the patient remains infection free; and the patient understands and complies with the medication regimen.

DOCUMENTATION
Guidelines

Document the administration of the medication immediately after administration, including date, time, dose, route of administration, site of administration, and rate of administration on the CMAR/MAR or record using the required format. If using a bar-code system, medication administration is automatically recorded when the bar code is scanned. PRN medications require documentation of the reason for administration. Prompt recording avoids the possibility of accidentally repeating the administration of the drug. If the drug was refused or omitted, record this in the appropriate area on the medication record and notify the primary care provider. This verifies the reason medication was omitted and ensures that the primary care provider is aware of the patient's condition. Document the volume of fluid administered on the intake and output record, if necessary.

UNEXPECTED SITUATIONS AND ASSOCIATED INTERVENTIONS

- *Upon assessing the IV site before administering medication, you note that the IV has infiltrated:* Stop IV fluid and remove the IV from the extremity. Restart the IV in a different location. Continue to monitor the new IV site as medication is administered.
- *While administering medication, you note a cloudy, white substance forming in the IV tubing:* Stop the IV from flowing and stop administering the medication to prevent precipitate from entering the patient's circulation. Clamp the IV at the site nearest to the patient. Replace tubing on primary and secondary infusions. Check the literature regarding incompatibilities of medications before administering. Medication infusion may require a second IV site or flushing of tubing before and after administration.
- *While you are administering medication, the patient begins to complain of pain at the IV site:* Stop the medication. Assess the IV site for any signs of infiltration or phlebitis. Flush the IV with normal saline to check for patency. If the IV site appears within normal limits, resume medication administration at a slower rate.

SPECIAL CONSIDERATIONS

General Considerations

• Ongoing assessment is an important part of nursing care for both evaluation of patient response to administered medications and early detection of adverse effects. If an adverse effect is suspected, withhold further medication doses and notify the patient's primary care provider. Additional intervention is based on type of reaction and patient assessment.

Infant and Child Considerations

• Infants and small children with fluid restrictions may not tolerate the added IV fluid needed for administration with piggyback or volume-control systems. For these children, consider using the mini-infusion pump.

SKILL 13 ADMINISTERING AN INTERMITTENT INTRAVENOUS INFUSION OF MEDICATION VIA A VOLUME-CONTROL ADMINISTRATION SET

With intermittent IV infusion, the drug is mixed with a small amount of the IV solution (e.g., 50 to 100 mL) and administered over a short period at the prescribed interval (e.g., every 4 hours). The administration is most often performed using an IV infusion pump, which requires the nurse to program the infusion rate into the pump. "Smart (computerized) pumps" are being used by many facilities for IV infusions, including intermittent infusions. Smart pumps also require programming of infusion rates by the nurse, but also are able to identify dosing limits and practice guidelines to aid in safe administration. Administration may also be achieved by gravity infusion, which requires the nurse to calculate the infusion rate in drops per minute. The best practice, however, is to use an intravenous infusion pump.

This skill discusses using a volume-control administration set for intermittent IV infusion. The medication is diluted with a small amount of solution and administered through the patient's IV line. This type of equipment may be used for infusing solutions into children, critically ill patients, and older patients when the fluid volume to be infused is a concern. Needleless devices (recommended by the CDC and the Occupational Safety and Health Administration [OSHA]) prevent needlesticks and provide access to the primary venous line. Either a blunt-ended cannula or a recessed connection port may be used to connect intermittent IV infusions.

DELEGATION CONSIDERATIONS

The administration of medications by intermittent IV infusion is not delegated to nursing assistive personnel (NAP) or to unlicensed assistive personnel (UAP). Depending on the state's nurse practice act and the organization's policies and procedures, the administration of specified IV medications in some settings may be delegated to licensed practical/vocational nurses (LPN/LVNs) who have received appropriate training. The decision to delegate must be based on careful analysis of the patient's needs and circumstances, as well as the qualifications of the person to whom the task is being delegated.

EQUIPMENT

• Prescribed medication
• Syringe with a needless device or blunt needle, if required, based on facility system
• Volume-control set (Volutrol, Buretrol, Burette)
• Needleless connector or stopcock, if required
• Infusion pump, if needed
• Antimicrobial swab
• Date label for tubing
• Medication label

(*continued*)

SKILL 13 ADMINISTERING AN INTERMITTENT INTRAVENOUS INFUSION OF MEDICATION VIA A VOLUME-CONTROL ADMINISTRATION SET continued

- Computer-generated Medication Administration Record (CMAR) or Medication Administration Record (MAR)
- PPE, as indicated

ASSESSMENT

Assess the patient for any allergies. Check the expiration date before administering the medication. Assess the appropriateness of the drug for the patient. Assess the compatibility of the ordered medication, diluent, and the infusing IV fluid. Review assessment and laboratory data that may influence drug administration. Assess the patient's knowledge of the medication. If the patient has a knowledge deficit about the medication, this may be the appropriate time to begin education about the medication. If the medication may affect the patient's vital signs, assess them before administration. Assess the IV insertion site, noting any swelling, coolness, leakage of fluid at site, redness, or pain.

NURSING DIAGNOSIS

Determine related factors for the nursing diagnoses based on the patient's current status. Appropriate nursing diagnoses include:

- Risk for Allergy Response
- Risk for Infection
- Risk for Injury

OUTCOME IDENTIFICATION AND PLANNING

The expected outcome to achieve when administering an intermittent IV infusion of medication via a volume-control set is that the medication is delivered via the IV route using sterile technique. Other outcomes that may be appropriate include the following: medication is delivered to the patient in a safe manner and at the appropriate infusion rate; the patient experiences no allergy response; the patient remains infection free; and the patient understands and complies with the medication regimen.

IMPLEMENTATION

ACTION	RATIONALE
1. Gather equipment. Check the medication order against the original order in the medical record according to facility policy. Clarify any inconsistencies. Check the patient's chart for allergies. Verify the compatibility of the medication and IV fluid.	This comparison helps to identify errors that may have occurred when orders were transcribed. The primary care provider's order is the legal record of medication orders for each facility.
2. Know the actions, special nursing considerations, safe dose ranges, purpose of administration, and adverse effects of the medications to be administered. Consider the appropriateness of the medication for this patient.	This knowledge aids the nurse in evaluating the therapeutic effect of the medication in relation to the patient's disorder and can also be used to educate the patient about the medication.
3. Perform hand hygiene.	Hand hygiene prevents the spread of microorganisms.
4. Move the medication cart to the outside of the patient's room or prepare for administration in the medication area.	Organization facilitates error-free administration and saves time.
5. Unlock the medication cart or drawer. Enter pass code and scan employee identification, if required.	Locking the cart or drawer safeguards each patient's medication supply. Hospital accrediting organizations require medication carts to be locked when not in use. Entering pass code and scanning ID allows only authorized users into the computer system and identifies the user for documentation by the computer.
6. **Prepare medication for one patient at a time.**	This prevents errors in medication administration.
7. Read the CMAR/MAR and select the proper medication from unit stock or the patient's medication drawer.	This is the *first* check of the label.

ACTION	RATIONALE
8. Compare the label with the CMAR/MAR. Check expiration dates and perform calculations, if necessary. Confirm the prescribed or appropriate infusion rate. Calculate the drip rate if using a gravity system. Scan the bar code on the package, if required. Check the infusion rate.	This is the *second* check of the label. Verify calculations with another nurse to ensure safety, if necessary. Delivers the correct dose of medication as prescribed.
9. If necessary, withdraw medication from an ampule or vial as described in Skills 3 and 4. Attach needleless connector or blunt needle to end of syringe, if necessary.	Allows for entry into the volume-control administration set chamber.
10. **Depending on facility policy, the third check of the label may occur at this point. If so, when all medications for one patient have been prepared, recheck the label with the CMAR/MAR before taking the medications to the patient.**	This *third* check ensures accuracy and helps to prevent errors. *Note:* Many facilities require the *third* check to occur at the bedside, after identifying the patient and before administration.
11. Prepare medication label, including name of medication, dose, total volume, including diluent, and time of administration.	Allows for accurate identification of medication.
12. Lock the medication cart before leaving it.	Locking the cart or drawer safeguards the patient's medication supply. Hospital accrediting organizations require medication carts to be locked when not in use.
13. Transport medications and equipment to the patient's bedside carefully, and keep the medications in sight at all times.	Careful handling and close observation prevent accidental or deliberate disarrangement of medications. Having equipment available saves time and facilitates performance of the task.
14. **Ensure that the patient receives the medications at the correct time.**	Check facility policy, which may allow for administration within a period of 30 minutes before or 30 minutes after the designated time.
15. Perform hand hygiene and put on PPE, if indicated.	Hand hygiene and PPE prevent the spread of microorganisms. PPE is required based on transmission precautions.
16. **Identify the patient. Compare the information with the CMAR/MAR. The patient should be identified using at least two methods** (The Joint Commission, 2013):	Identifying the patient ensures the right patient receives the medications and helps prevent errors. The patient's room number or physical location is not used as an identifier (The Joint Commission, 2013). Replace the identification band if it is missing or inaccurate in any way.
a. Check the name on the patient's identification band.	
b. Check the identification number on the patient's identification band.	
c. Check the birth date on the patient's identification band.	
d. Ask the patient to state his or her name and birth date, based on facility policy.	This requires a response from the patient, but illness and strange surroundings often cause patients to be confused.
17. Close the door to the room or pull the bedside curtain.	This provides patient privacy.
18. **Complete necessary assessments before administering medications. Check the patient's allergy bracelet or ask the patient about allergies. Explain the purpose and action of the medication to the patient.**	Assessment is a prerequisite to administration of medications. Explanation provides rationale, increases knowledge, and reduces anxiety.

(continued)

SKILL 13 ADMINISTERING AN INTERMITTENT INTRAVENOUS INFUSION OF MEDICATION VIA A VOLUME-CONTROL ADMINISTRATION SET continued

ACTION

19. Scan the patient's bar code on the identification band, if required (Figure 1).

20. **Based on facility policy, the third check of the label may occur at this point. If so, recheck the labels with the CMAR/MAR before administering the medications to the patient.**

21. Assess IV site for presence of inflammation or infiltration.

22. Fill the volume-control administration set (Figure 2) with the prescribed amount of IV fluid by opening the clamp between IV solution and the volume-control administration set. Follow manufacturer's instructions and fill with prescribed amount of IV solution (Figure 3). Close clamp.

RATIONALE

Provides an additional check to ensure that the medication is given to the right patient.

Many facilities require the *third* check to occur at the bedside, after identifying the patient and before administration. If facility policy directs the *third* check at this time, this *third* check ensures accuracy and helps to prevent errors.

IV medication must be given directly into a vein for safe administration.

This dilutes the medication in a minimal amount of solution. Reclamping prevents the continued addition of fluid to the volume to be mixed with the medication.

FIGURE 1 Scanning bar code on the patient's identification bracelet. *(Photo by B. Proud.)*

FIGURE 2 Volume-control administration set and IV solution for dilution of medication. *(Photo by B. Proud.)*

FIGURE 3 Opening clamp between IV solution and volume-control administration set to fill chamber with prescribed amount of solution. *(Photo by B. Proud.)*

ACTION	RATIONALE
23. Check to ensure the air vent on the volume-control administration set chamber is open.	Air vent allows fluid in the chamber to flow at a regular rate.
24. Use an antimicrobial swab to clean the access port on the volume-control administration set chamber (Figure 4).	This deters entry of microorganisms when the syringe enters the chamber.
25. Attach the syringe with a twisting motion into the access port while holding the syringe steady (Figure 5). Alternately, insert the needleless device or blunt needle into the port. Inject the medication into the chamber (Figure 6). Gently rotate the chamber.	This ensures that medication is evenly mixed with the solution.

FIGURE 4 Cleaning access port. *(Photo by B. Proud.)*

FIGURE 5 Attaching syringe to access port. *(Photo by B. Proud.)*

FIGURE 6 Injecting medication into chamber. *(Photo by B. Proud.)*

ACTION	RATIONALE
26. Attach the medication label to the volume-control device.	This identifies contents of the set and prevents medication error.
27. Use an antimicrobial swab to clean the access port or stopcock below the roller clamp on the primary IV infusion tubing, usually the port closest to the IV insertion site.	This deters entry of microorganisms when the piggyback setup is connected to the port. Proper connection allows IV medication to flow into primary line.
28. Connect the secondary infusion to the primary infusion at the cleansed port.	This allows for delivery of medication.
29. The volume-control administration set may be placed on an infusion pump with the appropriate dose programmed into the pump. Alternately, use the roller clamp on the volume-control administration set tubing to adjust the infusion to the prescribed rate.	Delivery over a 30- to 60-minute interval is a safe method of administering IV medication.
30. Discard the syringe in the appropriate receptacle.	Proper disposal prevents injury.
31. Clamp tubing on secondary set when solution is infused. Remove secondary tubing from access port and cap or replace connector with a new, capped one, if reusing. Follow facility policy regarding disposal of equipment.	Many facilities allow reuse of tubing for 48 to 96 hours. Replacing connector or needle with a new, capped one maintains sterility of system.
32. Check rate of primary infusion.	Administration of a secondary infusion may interfere with the primary infusion rate.
33. Remove PPE, if used. Perform hand hygiene.	Removing PPE properly reduces the risk for infection transmission and contamination of other items. Hand hygiene prevents the spread of microorganisms.

(continued)

SKILL 13 ADMINISTERING AN INTERMITTENT INTRAVENOUS INFUSION OF MEDICATION VIA A VOLUME-CONTROL ADMINISTRATION SET continued

ACTION	RATIONALE
34. Document the administration of the medication immediately after administration. See Documentation section below. Document the volume of fluid administered on the intake and output record, if necessary.	Timely documentation helps to ensure patient safety.
35. Evaluate the patient's response to the medication within appropriate time frame. Monitor IV site at periodic intervals.	The patient needs to be evaluated for therapeutic and adverse effects from the medication. Visualization of the site also allows for assessment of any untoward effects.

EVALUATION

The expected outcomes are met when the medication is delivered via the IV route using sterile technique; the medication is delivered to the patient in a safe manner and at the appropriate infusion rate; the patient experiences no allergy response; the patient remains infection free; and the patient understands and complies with the medication regimen.

DOCUMENTATION

Guidelines

Document the administration of the medication immediately after administration, including date, time, dose, route of administration, site of administration, and rate of administration on the CMAR/MAR or record using the required format. If using a bar-code system, medication administration is automatically recorded when bar code is scanned. PRN medications require documentation of the reason for administration. Prompt recording avoids the possibility of accidentally repeating the administration of the drug. If the drug was refused or omitted, record this in the appropriate area on the medication record and notify the primary care provider. This verifies the reason medication was omitted and ensures that the primary care provider is aware of the patient's condition. Document the volume of fluid administered on the intake and output record, if necessary.

UNEXPECTED SITUATIONS AND ASSOCIATED INTERVENTIONS

- *Upon assessing the IV site before administering the medication, you note that the IV has infiltrated:* Stop IV fluid and remove the IV from the extremity. Restart the IV in a different location. Continue to monitor the new IV site as medication is administered.
- *While administering the medication, you note a cloudy, white substance forming in the IV tubing:* Stop the IV from flowing and stop administering the medication to prevent precipitate from entering the patient's circulation. Clamp the IV at the site nearest to the patient. Replace tubing on primary and secondary infusions. Check the literature regarding incompatibilities of medications before administering. Medication infusion may require a second IV site or flushing of tubing before and after administration.
- *While you are administering the medication, the patient begins to complain of pain at the IV site:* Stop the medication. Assess the IV site for any signs of infiltration or phlebitis. Flush the IV with normal saline to check for patency. If the IV site appears within normal limits, resume medication administration at a slower rate.

SPECIAL CONSIDERATIONS

General Considerations

- Ongoing assessment is an important part of nursing care for both evaluation of patient response to administered medications and early detection of adverse effects. If an adverse effect is suspected, withhold further medication doses and notify the patient's primary care provider. Additional intervention is based on type of reaction and patient assessment.

Infant and Child Considerations

- Infants and small children with fluid restrictions may not tolerate the added IV fluid needed for administration with piggyback or volume-control systems. For these children, consider using a mini-infusion pump (Skill 12).

SKILL 14

INTRODUCING DRUGS THROUGH A MEDICATION OR DRUG-INFUSION LOCK (INTERMITTENT PERIPHERAL VENOUS ACCESS DEVICE) USING THE SALINE FLUSH

A medication or drug-infusion lock, also known as an intermittent peripheral venous access device, is used for patients who require intermittent IV medication, but not a continuous IV infusion. This device consists of a needle or catheter connected to a short length of tubing capped with a sealed injection port. After the catheter is in place in the patient's vein, the catheter and tubing are anchored to the patient's arm so that the catheter remains in place until the patient no longer requires the repeated medication intravenously.

The device is kept patent (working) by flushing with small amounts of saline pushed through the device on a routine basis. Using saline eliminates any possible systemic effects on coagulation, development of a heparin allergy, and drug incompatibility, which may occur when a heparin solution is used. The nurse must confirm IV placement before administration of medication. It is important to flush the drug-infusion lock before and after the medication is administered to clear the vein of any medication and to prevent clot formation in the device. If infiltration or phlebitis occurs, the lock is removed and replaced in a new site.

DELEGATION CONSIDERATIONS

The administration of medications through an intermittent peripheral venous access device is not delegated to nursing assistive personnel (NAP) or to unlicensed assistive personnel (UAP). Depending on the state's nurse practice act and the organization's policies and procedures, the administration of specified IV medications in some settings may be delegated to licensed practical/vocational nurses (LPN/LVNs) who have received appropriate training. The decision to delegate must be based on careful analysis of the patient's needs and circumstances, as well as the qualifications of the person to whom the task is being delegated.

EQUIPMENT

- Medication
- Saline flushes (2), volume according to facility policy, usually 2 to 3 mL
- Antimicrobial swabs
- Watch with second hand or stopwatch feature
- Disposable gloves
- Computer-generated Medication Administration Record (CMAR) or Medication Administration Record (MAR)

ASSESSMENT

Assess the patient for any allergies. Check the expiration date before administering the medication. Assess the appropriateness of the drug for the patient. Review assessment and laboratory data that may influence drug administration. Assess the patient's IV site, noting any swelling, coolness, leakage of fluid from IV site, or pain. Assess the patient's knowledge of the medication. If the patient has a knowledge deficit about the medication, this may be the appropriate time to begin education about the medication. If the medication may affect the patient's vital signs, assess them before administration. If the medication is for pain relief, assess the patient's pain before and after administration.

NURSING DIAGNOSIS

Determine related factors for the nursing diagnoses based on the patient's current status. Appropriate nursing diagnoses may include:

- Risk for Allergy Response
- Risk for Infection
- Deficient Knowledge

OUTCOME IDENTIFICATION AND PLANNING

The expected outcome to achieve when administering medication via a medication or drug-infusion lock is that the medication is delivered via the IV route using sterile technique. Other outcomes that may be appropriate include the following: medication is delivered to the patient in a safe manner and at the appropriate infusion rate; the patient experiences no adverse effect; and the patient understands and complies with the medication regimen.

(continued)

SKILL 14 | INTRODUCING DRUGS THROUGH A MEDICATION OR DRUG-INFUSION LOCK (INTERMITTENT PERIPHERAL VENOUS ACCESS DEVICE) USING THE SALINE FLUSH continued

IMPLEMENTATION

ACTION

1. Gather equipment. Check the medication order against the original order in the medical record, according to agency policy. Clarify any inconsistencies. Check the patient's chart for allergies. Check a drug resource to clarify whether medication needs to be diluted before administration. Verify the recommended administration rate.

2. Know the actions, special nursing considerations, safe dose ranges, purpose of administration, and adverse effects of the medications to be administered. Consider the appropriateness of the medication for this patient.

 3. Perform hand hygiene.

4. Move the medication cart to the outside of the patient's room or prepare for administration in the medication area.

5. Unlock the medication cart or drawer. Enter pass code and scan employee identification, if required.

6. **Prepare medication for one patient at a time.**

7. Read the CMAR/MAR and select the proper medication from unit stock or the patient's medication drawer.

8. Compare the label with the CMAR/MAR. Check expiration dates and perform calculations, if necessary. Scan the bar code on the package, if required.

9. If necessary, withdraw medication from an ampule or vial as described in Skills 3 and 4.

10. **Depending on facility policy, the third check of the label may occur at this point. If so, when all medications for one patient have been prepared, recheck the labels with the CMAR/MAR before taking the medications to the patient.**

11. Lock the medication cart before leaving it.

12. Transport medications and equipment to the patient's bedside carefully, and keep the medications in sight at all times.

13. **Ensure that the patient receives the medications at the correct time.**

RATIONALE

This comparison helps to identify errors that may have occurred when orders were transcribed. The primary care provider's order is the legal record of medication orders for each facility. Compatibility of medication and solution prevents complications. Recommended infusion rate delivers the correct dose of medication as prescribed.

This knowledge aids the nurse in evaluating the therapeutic effect of the medication in relation to the patient's disorder and can also be used to educate the patient about the medication.

Hand hygiene prevents the spread of microorganisms.

Organization facilitates error-free administration and saves time.

Locking the cart or drawer safeguards each patient's medication supply. Hospital accrediting organizations require medication carts to be locked when not in use. Entering pass code and scanning ID allows only authorized users into the system and identifies the user for documentation by the computer.

This prevents errors in medication administration.

This is the *first* check of the label.

This is the *second* check of the label. Verify calculations with another nurse to ensure safety, if necessary.

Allows administration of medication.

This *third* check ensures accuracy and helps to prevent errors. *Note:* Many facilities require the *third* check to occur at the bedside, after identifying the patient and before administration.

Locking the cart or drawer safeguards the patient's medication supply. Hospital accrediting organizations require medication carts to be locked when not in use.

Careful handling and close observation prevent accidental or deliberate disarrangement of medications. Having equipment available saves time and facilitates performance of the task.

Check facility policy, which may allow for administration within a period of 30 minutes before or 30 minutes after the designated time.

ACTION	RATIONALE

14. Perform hand hygiene and put on PPE, if indicated.

Hand hygiene and PPE prevent the spread of microorganisms. PPE is required based on transmission precautions.

15. **Identify the patient. Compare the information with the CMAR/MAR. The patient should be identified using at least two methods (The Joint Commission, 2013):**

Identifying the patient ensures the right patient receives the medications and helps prevent errors. The patient's room number or physical location is not used as an identifier (The Joint Commission, 2013). Replace the identification band if it is missing or inaccurate in any way.

   a. Check the name on the patient's identification band.

   b. Check the identification number on the patient's identification band.

   c. Check the birth date on the patient's identification band.

   d. Ask the patient to state his or her name and birth date, based on facility policy.

This requires a response from the patient, but illness and strange surroundings often cause patients to be confused.

16. Close the door to the room or pull the bedside curtain.

This provides patient privacy.

17. **Complete necessary assessments before administering medications. Check the patient's allergy bracelet or ask the patient about allergies. Explain the purpose and action of the medication to the patient.**

Assessment is a prerequisite to administration of medications. Explanation provides rationale, increases knowledge, and reduces anxiety.

18. Scan the patient's bar code on the identification band, if required (Figure 1).

Scanning provides an additional check to ensure that the medication is given to the right patient.

19. **Based on facility policy, the third check of the label may occur at this point. If so, recheck the labels with the CMAR/MAR before administering the medications to the patient.**

Many facilities require the *third* check to occur at the bedside, after identifying the patient and before administration. If facility policy directs the *third* check at this time, this *third* check ensures accuracy and helps to prevent errors.

20. Assess IV site for presence of inflammation or infiltration.

IV medication must be given directly into a vein for safe administration.

21. Put on clean gloves.

Gloves protect the nurse's hands from contact with the patient's blood.

22. Clean the access port of the medication lock with antimicrobial swab (Figure 2).

Cleaning removes surface contaminants at the lock entry site.

FIGURE 1 Scanning bar code on patient's identification bracelet.

FIGURE 2 Cleaning access port.

(continued)

SKILL 14 INTRODUCING DRUGS THROUGH A MEDICATION OR DRUG-INFUSION LOCK (INTERMITTENT PERIPHERAL VENOUS ACCESS DEVICE) USING THE SALINE FLUSH continued

ACTION	RATIONALE
23. Stabilize the port with your nondominant hand and insert the syringe, or needleless access device, of normal saline into the access port (Figure 3).	This allows for careful insertion into the center circle of the lock.
24. Release the clamp on the extension tubing of the medication lock. Aspirate gently and check for blood return (Figure 4).	This ensures the catheter of the medication lock is in a vein.

FIGURE 3 Inserting syringe into access port.

FIGURE 4 Aspirating for blood return.

25. Gently flush with normal saline by pushing slowly on the syringe plunger. Observe the insertion site while inserting the saline. Remove syringe.	Saline flush ensures that the IV line is patent. Puffiness or swelling as the site is flushed could indicate infiltration of the catheter.
26. Insert syringe, or needleless access device, with medication into the port and gently inject medication, using a watch to verify correct administration rate. **Do not force the injection if resistance is felt.**	Easy installation of medication usually indicates that the lock is still patent and in the vein. If force is used against resistance, a clot may break away and cause a blockage elsewhere in the body.
27. Remove the medication syringe from the port. Stabilize the port with your nondominant hand and insert the syringe, or needleless access device, of normal saline into the port. Gently flush with normal saline by pushing slowly on the syringe plunger (Figure 5). If the medication lock is capped with positive pressure valve/device, remove syringe, and then clamp the extension tubing (Figure 6). Alternately, to gain positive pressure if positive pressure valve/device is not present, clamp the extension tubing as you are still flushing the last of the saline into the medication lock. Remove syringe.	Positive pressure prevents blood from backing into the catheter and causing the medication lock to clot off.

FIGURE 5 Flushing port with normal saline.

FIGURE 6 Clamping access port.

ACTION	**RATIONALE**
28. Discard the syringe in the appropriate receptacle.	Proper disposal prevents injury.
29. Remove PPE, if used. Perform hand hygiene.	Removing PPE properly reduces the risk for infection transmission and contamination of other items. Hand hygiene prevents the spread of microorganisms.
30. Document the administration of the medication immediately after administration. See Documentation section below.	Timely documentation helps to ensure patient safety.
31. Evaluate the patient's response to the medication within an appropriate time frame.	The patient needs to be evaluated for therapeutic and adverse effects from the medication.
32. Check the medication lock site at least every 8 hours or according to facility policy.	This ensures patency of system.

EVALUATION

The expected outcomes are met when the medication is delivered via the IV route using sterile technique; the medication is delivered to the patient in a safe manner and at the appropriate infusion rate; the patient experiences no adverse effect; the intermittent peripheral venous access device remains patent; and the patient understands and complies with the medication regimen.

DOCUMENTATION

Guidelines

Document the administration of the medication and saline flush, including date, time, dose, route of administration, site of administration, and rate of administration on the CMAR/MAR or record using the required format, immediately after administration. If using a bar-code system, medication administration is automatically recorded when the bar code is scanned. PRN medications require documentation of the reason for administration. Prompt recording avoids the possibility of accidentally repeating the administration of the drug. If the drug was refused or omitted, record this in the appropriate area on the medication record and notify the primary care provider. This verifies the reason medication was omitted and ensures that the primary care provider is aware of the patient's condition.

UNEXPECTED SITUATIONS AND ASSOCIATED INTERVENTIONS

- *Upon assessing the medication lock site before administering the medication, you note that the medication lock has infiltrated:* Remove the medication lock from the extremity. Restart peripheral venous access in a different location. Continue to monitor the new site as medication is administered.
- *While you are administering medication, the patient begins to complain of pain at the site:* Stop the medication. Assess the medication lock site for signs of infiltration and phlebitis. Flush the medication lock with normal saline again to recheck patency. If the IV site appears within normal limits, resume medication administration at a slower rate. If pain persists, stop, remove medication lock and restart in a different location.
- *As you are attempting to access the lock, the syringe tip touches the patient's arm:* Discard syringe. Prepare a new dose for administration.
- *No blood return is noted upon aspiration:* If the medication lock appears patent, without signs of infiltration, and normal saline fluid infuses without difficulty, proceed with administration. Observe closely for signs and symptoms of infiltration during and after administration.

SPECIAL CONSIDERATIONS

General Considerations

- If a medication lock is not used, flush with saline every 8 to 12 hours to maintain patency, according to facility policy.
- Routinely change the medication lock site every 72 to 96 hours, according to facility policy. This reduces the risk of infection and emboli in the bloodstream.

(continued)

SKILL 14

INTRODUCING DRUGS THROUGH A MEDICATION OR DRUG-INFUSION LOCK (INTERMITTENT PERIPHERAL VENOUS ACCESS DEVICE) USING THE SALINE FLUSH continued

- Intermittent infusions of small-volume IV medications can also be administered through the medication lock. Attach IV medication container to infusion tubing and prime. After flushing the medication lock with saline as outlined above, attach the infusion tubing to the medication lock. Set the infusion rate in the infusion pump. Alternately, adjust the infusion rate with the roller clamp on the gravity infusion tubing. After infusion is completed, remove tubing from the lock and flush with saline as outlined above.
- Ongoing assessment is an important part of nursing care to evaluate patient response to administered medications and early detection of adverse effects. If an adverse effect is suspected, withhold further medication doses and notify the patient's primary care provider. Additional intervention is based on type of reaction and patient assessment.

Infant and Child Considerations

- If the volume of medication being administered is small (less than 1.0 mL), always include the amount of flush solution as part of the total amount to be injected and take this into account when determining how fast to push a medication. For example, if the medication is to be injected at a rate of 1.0 mL per minute and the total amount of solution to be injected is 2.25 mL (0.25 mL medication volume plus 2.0 mL saline flush solution volume equals 2.25 mL), then the medication would be injected over a period of 2 minutes 15 seconds.

SKILL 15 | INSTILLING EYE DROPS

Eye drops are instilled for their local effects, such as for pupil dilation or constriction when examining the eye, for infection treatment, or for controlling intraocular pressure (for patients with glaucoma). The type and amount of solution administered depends on the purpose of the instillation.

The eye is a delicate organ, highly susceptible to infection and injury. Although the eye is never free of microorganisms, the secretions of the conjunctiva protect against many pathogens. For maximal safety for the patient, the equipment, solutions, and ointments introduced into the conjunctival sac should be sterile. If this is not possible, follow careful guidelines for medical asepsis.

Refer to the accompanying Skill Variation for the steps to administer eye ointment.

DELEGATION CONSIDERATIONS

The administration of medication via drops in the eye is not delegated to nursing assistive personnel (NAP) or to unlicensed assistive personnel (UAP). Depending on the state's nurse practice act and the organization's policies and procedures, the administration of eye drops may be delegated to licensed practical/vocational nurses (LPN/LVNs). The decision to delegate must be based on careful analysis of the patient's needs and circumstances, as well as the qualifications of the person to whom the task is being delegated.

EQUIPMENT

- Gloves
- Additional PPE, as indicated
- Medication
- Tissues
- Normal saline solution
- Washcloth, cotton balls, or gauze squares
- Computer-generated Medication Administration Record (CMAR) or Medication Administration Record (MAR)

ASSESSMENT

Assess the patient for any allergies. Check the expiration date before administering the medication. Assess the appropriateness of the drug for the patient. Review assessment and laboratory data that may influence drug administration. Verify patient name, dose, route, and time of administration. Assess the affected eye for any drainage, erythema, or swelling. Assess the patient's knowledge of the medication. If the patient has a knowledge deficit about the medication, this may be the appropriate time to begin education about the medication. If the medication may affect the patient's vital signs, assess them before administration.

NURSING DIAGNOSIS

Determine related factors for the nursing diagnoses based on the patient's current status. Appropriate nursing diagnoses may include:

- Risk for Allergy Response
- Deficient Knowledge
- Risk for Injury

OUTCOME IDENTIFICATION AND PLANNING

The expected outcome to achieve when administering eye drops is that the medication is delivered successfully into the eye. Other outcomes that may be appropriate include the following: the patient experiences no allergy response; the patient does not exhibit systemic effects of the medication; the patient's eye remains free from injury; and patient understands the rationale for medication administration.

IMPLEMENTATION

ACTION

1. Gather equipment. Check medication order against the original order in the medical record, according to facility policy. Clarify any inconsistencies. Check the patient's chart for allergies.

2. Know the actions, special nursing considerations, safe dose ranges, purpose of administration, and adverse effects of the medications to be administered. Consider the appropriateness of the medication for this patient.

3. Perform hand hygiene.

4. Move the medication cart to the outside of the patient's room or prepare for administration in the medication area.

5. Unlock the medication cart or drawer. Enter pass code and scan employee identification, if required.

6. **Prepare medications for one patient at a time.**

7. Read the CMAR/MAR and select the proper medication from the patient's medication drawer or unit stock.

8. Compare the label with the CMAR/MAR. Check expiration dates and perform calculations, if necessary. Scan the bar code on the package, if required.

RATIONALE

This comparison helps to identify errors that may have occurred when orders were transcribed. The primary care provider's order is the legal record of medication orders for each facility.

This knowledge aids the nurse in evaluating the therapeutic effect of the medication in relation to the patient's disorder and can also be used to educate the patient about the medication.

Hand hygiene prevents the spread of microorganisms.

Organization facilitates error-free administration and saves time.

Locking the cart or drawer safeguards each patient's medication supply. Hospital accrediting organizations require medication carts to be locked when not in use. Entering pass code and scanning ID allows only authorized users into the system and identifies the user for documentation by the computer.

This prevents errors in medication administration.

This is the *first* check of the label.

This is the *second* check of the label. Verify calculations with another nurse to ensure safety, if necessary.

(continued)

SKILL 15 INSTILLING EYE DROPS continued

ACTION	RATIONALE

ACTION

9. Depending on facility policy, the third check of the label may occur at this point. If so, when all medications for one patient have been prepared, recheck the labels with the CMAR/MAR before taking the medications to the patient.

10. Lock the medication cart before leaving it.

11. Transport medications to the patient's bedside carefully, and keep the medications in sight at all times.

12. Ensure that the patient receives the medications at the correct time.

13. Perform hand hygiene and put on PPE, if indicated.

14. Identify the patient. Compare the information with the CMAR/MAR. The patient should be identified using at least two methods (The Joint Commission, 2013):

a. Check the name on the patient's identification band.

b. Check the identification number on the patient's identification band.

c. Check the birth date on the patient's identification band.

d. Ask the patient to state his or her name and birth date, based on facility policy.

15. Complete necessary assessments before administering medications. Check the patient's allergy bracelet or ask the patient about allergies. Explain the purpose and action of each medication to the patient.

16. Scan the patient's bar code on the identification band, if required (Figure 1).

RATIONALE

This *third* check ensures accuracy and helps to prevent errors. *Note:* Many facilities require the *third* check to occur at the bedside, after identifying the patient and before administration.

Locking the cart or drawer safeguards the patient's medication supply. Hospital accrediting organizations require medication carts to be locked when not in use.

Careful handling and close observation prevent accidental or deliberate disarrangement of medications.

Check agency policy, which may allow for administration within a period of 30 minutes before or 30 minutes after the designated time.

Hand hygiene and PPE prevent the spread of microorganisms. PPE is required based on transmission precautions.

Identifying the patient ensures the right patient receives the medications and helps prevent errors. The patient's room number or physical location is not used as an identifier (The Joint Commission, 2013). Replace the identification band if it is missing or inaccurate in any way.

This requires a response from the patient, but illness and strange surroundings often cause patients to be confused.

Assessment is a prerequisite to administration of medications.

Provides an additional check to ensure that the medication is given to the right patient.

FIGURE 1 Scanning bar code on patient's identification bracelet.

ACTION

17. **Based on facility policy, the third check of the label may occur at this point. If so, recheck the labels with the CMAR/MAR before administering the medications to the patient.**

18. Put on gloves.

19. Offer tissue to patient.

20. Cleanse the eyelids and eyelashes of any drainage with a washcloth, cotton balls, or gauze squares moistened with normal saline solution. Use each area of the cleaning surface once, moving from the inner toward the outer canthus (Figure 2).

RATIONALE

Many facilities require the *third* check to occur at the bedside, after identifying the patient and before administration. If facility policy directs the *third* check at this time, this *third* check ensures accuracy and helps to prevent errors.

Gloves protect the nurse from potential contact with mucous membranes and body fluids.

Solution and tears may spill from the eye during the procedure.

Debris can be carried into the eye when the conjunctival sac is exposed. Using each area of the gauze once and moving from the inner canthus to the outer canthus prevents carrying debris to the lacrimal ducts.

FIGURE 2 Cleaning lids and lashes from inside of eye to outside.

21. Tilt the patient's head back slightly if sitting, or place the patient's head over a pillow if lying down. **Tilting the patient's head should be avoided if the patient has a cervical spine injury.** The head may be turned slightly to the affected side to prevent solution or tears from flowing toward the opposite eye (Figure 3).

Tilting the patient's head back slightly makes it easier to reach the conjunctival sac. Turning the head to the affected side helps to prevent solution or tears from flowing toward the opposite eye.

FIGURE 3 Turning head slightly to affected side.

(*continued*)

SKILL 15 INSTILLING EYE DROPS continued

ACTION	RATIONALE
22. Remove the cap from the medication bottle, being careful not to touch the inner side of the cap. (See the accompanying Skill Variation for administering ointment.)	Touching the inner side of the cap may contaminate the bottle of medication.
23. Invert the monodrip plastic container that is commonly used to instill eye drops. Have the patient look up and focus on something on the ceiling.	By having the patient look up and focus on something else, the procedure is less traumatic and keeps the eye still.
24. Place thumb or two fingers near margin of lower eyelid immediately below eyelashes, and exert pressure downward over bony cheek prominence. The lower conjunctival sac is exposed as the lower lid is pulled down (Figure 4).	The eye drop should be placed in the conjunctival sac, not directly on the eyeball.
25. **Hold the dropper close to the eye, but avoid touching eyelids or lashes.** Squeeze container and allow prescribed number of drops to fall in lower conjunctival sac (Figure 5).	Touching the eye, eyelids, or lashes can contaminate the medication in the bottle; startle the patient, causing blinking; or injure the eye. Do not allow medication to fall onto the cornea. This may injure the cornea or cause the patient to have an unpleasant sensation.

FIGURE 4 Exerting pressure downward to expose lower conjunctival sac.

FIGURE 5 Administering drops into conjunctival sac.

26. Release lower lid after eye drops are instilled. Ask patient to close eyes gently.	This allows the medication to be distributed over the entire eye.
27. Apply gentle pressure over inner canthus to prevent eye drops from flowing into tear duct (Figure 6).	This minimizes the risk of systemic effects from the medication.

FIGURE 6 Applying gentle pressure over inner canthus.

ACTION	RATIONALE
28. Instruct patient not to rub affected eye.	This prevents injury and irritation to the eye.
29. Remove gloves. Assist the patient to a comfortable position.	This ensures patient comfort.
30. Remove additional PPE, if used. Perform hand hygiene.	Removing PPE properly reduces the risk for infection transmission and contamination of other items. Hand hygiene prevents the spread of microorganisms.
31. Document the administration of the medication immediately after administration. See Documentation section below.	Timely documentation helps to ensure patient safety.
32. Evaluate the patient's response to the medication within an appropriate time frame.	The patient needs to be evaluated for therapeutic and adverse effects from the medication.

EVALUATION

The expected outcomes are met when the patient receives the eye drops; experiences no adverse effects, including allergy response, systemic effect, or injury; and understands the rationale for the medication administration.

DOCUMENTATION

Guidelines

Document the administration of the medication immediately after administration, including date, time, dose, route of administration, and site of administration, specifically right, left, or both eyes, on the CMAR/MAR or record using the required format. If using a bar-code system, medication administration is automatically recorded when the bar code is scanned. PRN medications require documentation of the reason for administration. Prompt recording avoids the possibility of accidentally repeating the administration of the drug. If the drug was refused or omitted, record this in the appropriate area on the medication record and notify the primary care provider. This verifies the reason medication was omitted and ensures that the primary care provider is aware of the patient's condition.

UNEXPECTED SITUATIONS AND ASSOCIATED INTERVENTIONS

- *Drop is placed on eyelid or outer margin of eyelid due to patient blinking or moving:* Do not count this drop in total number of drops administered. Allow the patient to regain composure and proceed with application of medication. Consider approaching the patient from below the line of sight.
- *You cannot open eyelids due to dried crust and matting of eyelids:* Place a warm, wet washcloth over the eye and allow it to remain there for approximately 3 minutes. Cleanse eye as described previously. You may need to repeat this procedure if there is a large amount of matting.
- *Bottle or tube of medication comes in contact with the eyeball when applying medication:* Bottle is contaminated; discard appropriately. Notify pharmacy or retrieve a new bottle for the oncoming shift.

SPECIAL CONSIDERATIONS

General Considerations

- Ongoing assessment is an important part of nursing care to evaluate patient response to administered medications and early detection of adverse effects. If an adverse effect is suspected, withhold further medication doses and notify the patient's primary care provider. Additional intervention is based on type of reaction and patient assessment.

Infant and Child Considerations

- To apply eye drops in a small child, two or more people may be needed to restrain the child. Make sure the child does not reach up to the eye, causing the nurse to jab the medication bottle into the eye.

(continued)

SKILL 15 | INSTILLING EYE DROPS   continued

SKILL VARIATION | Administering Eye Ointment

Prepare medication as outlined in steps 1–12 above (Skill 15).

1. Perform hand hygiene and put on PPE, if indicated.

2. Identify the patient. The patient should be identified using two methods.

3. Close the door to the room or pull the bedside curtain.
4. Complete necessary assessments before administering medications. Check allergy bracelet or ask patient about allergies. Explain the purpose and action of the medication to the patient.
5. Scan the patient's bar code on the identification band, if required.
6. Based on facility policy, the *third check* of the label may occur at this point. If so, recheck the labels with the CMAR/MAR before administering the medications to the patient.
7. Put on gloves. Offer the patient a tissue.
8. Cleanse the eyelids and eyelashes of any drainage with cotton balls or gauze squares moistened with normal saline solution. Use each area of the gauze square once, moving from the inner toward the outer canthus of the eye.
9. Tilt the patient's head back slightly if sitting, or place the patient's head over a pillow if lying down. The head may

be turned slightly to the affected side to prevent ointment or tears from flowing toward the opposite eye.
10. Have the patient look up and focus on something on the ceiling.
11. Place thumb or two fingers near margin of lower eyelid immediately below eyelashes and exert pressure downward over bony cheek prominence. Lower conjunctival sac is exposed as lower lid is pulled down.
12. Hold the ointment tube close to eye, but avoid touching eyelids or lashes. Squeeze container and apply about 0.5 inch of ointment from the tube along the exposed sac. Apply the medication, moving from the inner canthus to the outer canthus. Twist tube to break off ribbon of ointment. Do not touch the tip to the eye.
13. Release lower lid after ointment is instilled. Ask the patient to close eyes gently.
14. The warmth helps to liquefy the ointment. Instruct the patient to move the eye, because this helps to spread the ointment under the lids and over the surface of the eyeball.
15. Assist the patient to a comfortable position. Explain that the ointment may temporarily blur vision; encourage the patient not to rub the eye.
16. Remove gloves and additional PPE, if used. Perform hand hygiene.
17. Document administration of the medication on the CMAR/MAR immediately after administering the medication.
18. Evaluate the patient's response to the medication within an appropriate time frame.

SKILL 16 | INSTILLING EAR DROPS

Drugs are instilled into the auditory canal for their local effect. They are used to soften wax, relieve pain, apply local anesthesia, and treat infections.

The tympanic membrane separates the external ear from the middle ear. Normally, it is intact and closes the entrance to the middle ear completely. If it is ruptured or has been opened by surgical intervention, the middle ear and the inner ear have a direct passage to the external ear. When this occurs, perform instillations with the greatest of care to prevent forcing materials from the outer ear into the middle ear and the inner ear. Use sterile technique to prevent infection.

DELEGATION CONSIDERATIONS

The administration of medication via drops in the ear is not delegated to nursing assistive personnel (NAP) or to unlicensed assistive personnel (UAP). Depending on the state's nurse practice act and the organization's policies and procedures, the administration of ear drop may be delegated to licensed practical/vocational nurses (LPN/LVNs). The decision to delegate must be based on careful analysis of the patient's needs and circumstances, as well as the qualifications of the person to whom the task is being delegated.

EQUIPMENT	
	• Medication (warmed to 37°C [98.6°F])
	• Dropper
	• Tissue
	• Cotton balls (optional)
	• Gloves
	• Additional PPE, as indicated
	• Washcloth (optional)
	• Normal saline solution
	• Computer-generated Medication Administration Record (CMAR) or Medication Administration Record (MAR)

ASSESSMENT

Assess the affected ear for redness, erythema, edema, drainage, or tenderness. Assess the patient for allergies. Verify patient name, dose, route, and time of administration. Assess the patient's knowledge of medication and procedure. If the patient has a knowledge deficit about the medication, this may be an appropriate time to begin education about the medication. Assess the patient's ability to cooperate with the procedure.

NURSING DIAGNOSIS

Determine related factors for the nursing diagnoses based on the patient's current status. Appropriate nursing diagnoses may include:

- Anxiety
- Risk for Injury
- Acute Pain

OUTCOME IDENTIFICATION AND PLANNING

The expected outcome to achieve is that drops are administered successfully. Other outcomes that may be appropriate include the following: the patient understands the rationale for the ear drop instillation and has decreased anxiety; the patient remains free from pain; and the patient experiences no allergy response or injury.

IMPLEMENTATION

ACTION	RATIONALE
1. Gather equipment. Check medication order against the original order in the medical record, according to facility policy. Clarify any inconsistencies. Check the patient's chart for allergies.	This comparison helps to identify errors that may have occurred when orders were transcribed. The primary care provider's order is the legal record of medication orders for each facility.
2. Know the actions, special nursing considerations, safe dose ranges, purpose of administration, and adverse effects of the medication to be administered. Consider the appropriateness of the medication for this patient.	This knowledge aids the nurse in evaluating the therapeutic effect of the medication in relation to the patient's disorder and can also be used to educate the patient about the medication.
3. Perform hand hygiene.	Hand hygiene prevents the spread of microorganisms.
4. Move the medication cart to the outside of the patient's room or prepare for administration in the medication area.	Organization facilitates error-free administration and saves time.
5. Unlock the medication cart or drawer. Enter pass code and scan employee identification, if required.	Locking the cart or drawer safeguards each patient's medication supply. Hospital accrediting organizations require medication carts to be locked when not in use. Entering pass code and scanning ID allows only authorized users into the system and identifies the user for documentation by the computer.
6. **Prepare medications for one patient at a time.**	This prevents errors in medication administration.

(continued)

SKILL 16 INSTILLING EAR DROPS continued

ACTION	RATIONALE
7. Read the CMAR/MAR and select the proper medication from the patient's medication drawer or unit stock.	This is the *first* check of the label.
8. Compare the label with the CMAR/MAR. Check expiration dates and perform calculations, if necessary. Scan the bar code on the package, if required.	This is the *second* check of the label. Verify calculations with another nurse to ensure safety, if necessary.
9. Depending on facility policy, the third check of the label may occur at this point. If so, when all medications for one patient have been prepared, recheck the labels with the CMAR/MAR before taking the medications to the patient.	This *third* check ensures accuracy and helps to prevent errors. *Note:* Many facilities require the *third* check to occur at the bedside, after identifying the patient and before administration.
10. Lock the medication cart before leaving it.	Locking the cart or drawer safeguards the patient's medication supply. Hospital accrediting organizations require medication carts to be locked when not in use.
11. Transport medications to the patient's bedside carefully, and keep the medications in sight at all times.	Careful handling and close observation prevent accidental or deliberate disarrangement of medications.
12. Ensure that the patient receives the medications at the correct time.	Check agency policy, which may allow for administration within a period of 30 minutes before or 30 minutes after the designated time.
13. Perform hand hygiene and put on PPE, if indicated.	Hand hygiene and PPE prevent the spread of microorganisms. PPE is required based on transmission precautions.
14. Identify the patient. Compare the information with the CMAR/MAR. The patient should be identified using at least two methods (The Joint Commission, 2013):	Identifying the patient ensures the right patient receives the medications and helps prevent errors. The patient's room number or physical location is not used as an identifier (The Joint Commission, 2013). Replace the identification band if it is missing or inaccurate in any way.
a. Check the name on the patient's identification band.	
b. Check the identification number on the patient's identification band.	
c. Check the birth date on the patient's identification band.	
d. Ask the patient to state his or her name and birth date, based on facility policy.	This requires a response from the patient, but illness and strange surroundings often cause patients to be confused.
15. Complete necessary assessments before administering medications. Check the patient's allergy bracelet or ask the patient about allergies. Explain the purpose and action of each medication to the patient.	Assessment is a prerequisite to administration of medications.
16. Scan the patient's bar code on the identification band, if required.	Provides an additional check to ensure that the medication is given to the right patient.
17. Based on facility policy, the third check of the label may occur at this point. If so, recheck the labels with the CMAR/MAR before administering the medications to the patient.	Many facilities require the *third* check to occur at the bedside, after identifying the patient and before administration. If facility policy directs the *third* check at this time, this *third* check ensures accuracy and helps to prevent errors.
18. Put on gloves.	Gloves protect the nurse from potential contact with mucous membranes and body fluids.
19. Cleanse external ear of any drainage with cotton ball or washcloth moistened with normal saline (Figure 1).	Debris and drainage may prevent some of the medication from entering the ear canal.

ACTION

20. Place patient on his or her unaffected side in bed, or, if ambulatory, have patient sit with head well tilted to the side so that the affected ear is uppermost (Figure 2).

21. Draw up the amount of solution needed in the dropper. Do not return excess medication to stock bottle. A prepackaged, monodrip plastic container may also be used (Figure 3).

22. Straighten auditory canal by pulling cartilaginous portion of pinna up and back for an adult. (See Infant and Child Considerations for correct positioning for this age group.)

23. Hold dropper in the ear with its tip above the auditory canal (Figure 4). Do not touch the dropper to the ear. For an infant or an irrational or confused patient, protect the dropper with a piece of soft tubing to help prevent injury to the ear.

RATIONALE

This positioning prevents the drops from escaping from the ear.

Risk for contamination is increased when medication is returned to the stock bottle.

Pulling on the pinna as described helps to straighten the canal properly for ear drop instillation.

By holding the dropper in the ear, most of the medication will enter the ear canal. Touching the dropper to the ear contaminates the dropper and medication. The hard tip of the dropper can damage the tympanic membrane if it is jabbed into the ear.

FIGURE 1 Cleaning external ear.

FIGURE 2 Positioning patient on unaffected side.

FIGURE 3 Prepackaged ear drop solution.

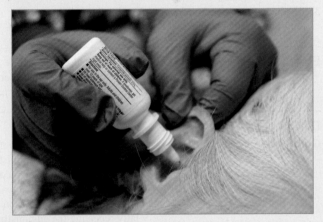

FIGURE 4 Pulling the pinna up and back and placing dropper tip above auditory canal.

24. **Allow drops to fall on the side of the canal. Avoid instilling in the middle of the canal, to avoid instilling directly onto the tympanic membrane.**

25. Release pinna after instilling drops, and have patient maintain the head position to prevent escape of medication.

It is uncomfortable for the patient if the drops fall directly onto the tympanic membrane.

Medication should remain in ear canal for at least 5 minutes.

(*continued*)

SKILL 16 INSTILLING EAR DROPS continued

ACTION	RATIONALE
26. Gently press on the tragus a few times (Figure 5).	Pressing on the tragus causes medication from the canal to move toward the tympanic membrane.
27. If ordered, loosely insert a cotton ball into the ear canal (Figure 6).	A cotton ball can help prevent medication from leaking out of the ear canal.

FIGURE 5 Applying pressure to tragus.

FIGURE 6 Inserting cotton ball into ear canal.

ACTION	RATIONALE
28. Remove gloves. Assist the patient to a comfortable position.	This ensures patient comfort.
29. Remove additional PPE, if used. Perform hand hygiene.	Removing PPE properly reduces the risk for infection transmission and contamination of other items. Hand hygiene prevents the spread of microorganisms.
30. Document the administration of the medication immediately after administration. See Documentation section below.	Timely documentation helps to ensure patient safety.
31. Evaluate the patient's response to medication within an appropriate time frame.	The patient needs to be evaluated for therapeutic and adverse effects from the medication.

EVALUATION

The expected outcomes are met when the patient receives the ear drops successfully; the patient understands the rationale for ear drop instillation and exhibits no or decreased anxiety; the patient experiences no or minimal pain and no allergy response or injury.

DOCUMENTATION

Guidelines

Document the administration of the medication immediately after administration, including date, time, dose, route of administration, and site of administration, specifically right, left, or both ears, on the CMAR/MAR or record using the required format. If using a bar-code system, medication administration is automatically recorded when the bar code is scanned. PRN medications require documentation of the reason for administration. Prompt recording avoids the possibility of accidentally repeating the administration of the drug. Document pre- and post-administration assessments, characteristics of any drainage, and the patient's response to the treatment, if appropriate. If the drug was refused or omitted, record this in the appropriate area on the medication record and notify the primary care provider. This verifies the reason medication was omitted and ensures that the primary care provider is aware of the patient's condition.

UNEXPECTED SITUATIONS AND ASSOCIATED INTERVENTIONS

- *Medication runs from ear into eye:* Notify primary care provider and check with the pharmacy. Eye irrigation may need to be performed.
- *Patient complains of extreme pain when you press on the tragus:* Allow patient to press on tragus. If pressure causes too much pain, this part may be deferred.

SPECIAL CONSIDERATIONS

General Considerations

- If both ears are to be treated, wait 5 minutes before instilling drops into the second ear.
- Ongoing assessment is an important part of nursing care to evaluate patient response to administered treatments and early detection of adverse effects. If an adverse effect is suspected, notify the patient's primary care provider. Additional intervention is based on type of reaction and patient assessment.

Infant and Child Considerations

- Pull pinna straight back for a child older than 3 years (Figure 7) and down and back for an infant or a child younger than 3 years (Figure 8).
- Distraction techniques, such as TV or a quiet toy, may be helpful when attempting to keep a child quiet for 5 minutes. Reading to the child may not be appropriate because the child's hearing may be compromised during medication administration.

FIGURE 7 Pulling pinna straight back for child older than 3 years.

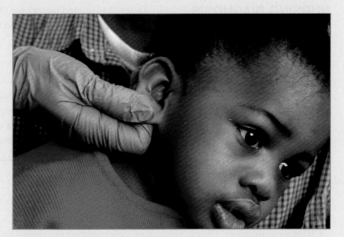

FIGURE 8 Pulling pinna down and back for an infant or child younger than 3 years.

SKILL 17   ADMINISTERING A NASAL SPRAY

Nasal instillations are used to treat allergies, sinus infections, and nasal congestion. Medications with a systemic effect, such as vasopressin, may also be prepared as a nasal instillation. The nose is normally not a sterile cavity, but because of its connection with the sinuses, it is important to observe medical asepsis carefully when using nasal instillations.

The following skill describes the steps to administer a nasal spray. Refer to the accompanying Skill Variation for guidelines to administer medication via nasal drops.

DELEGATION CONSIDERATIONS

The administration of medication using a nasal spray is not delegated to nursing assistive personnel (NAP) or to unlicensed assistive personnel (UAP). Depending on the state's nurse practice act and the organization's policies and procedures, administration of a nasal spray may be delegated to licensed practical/vocational nurses (LPN/LVNs). The decision to delegate must be based on careful analysis of the patient's needs and circumstances, as well as the qualifications of the person to whom the task is being delegated.

(continued)

SKILL 17 ADMINISTERING A NASAL SPRAY continued

EQUIPMENT	• Medication in nasal spray bottle • Gloves • Additional PPE, as indicated • Tissue • Computer-generated Medication Administration Record (CMAR) or Medication Administration Record (MAR)
ASSESSMENT	Assess the nares for redness, erythema, edema, drainage, or tenderness. Assess the patient for allergies. Verify patient name, dose, route, and time of administration. Assess the patient's knowledge of medication and the procedure. If the patient has a knowledge deficit about the medication, this may be an appropriate time to begin education about the procedure. Assess the patient's ability to cooperate with the procedure.
NURSING DIAGNOSIS	Determine related factors for the nursing diagnoses based on the patient's current status. Appropriate nursing diagnoses may include: • Deficient Knowledge • Risk for Allergy Response
OUTCOME IDENTIFICATION AND PLANNING	The expected outcome to achieve is that the medication is administered successfully into the nose. Other outcomes that may be appropriate include the following: the patient understands the rationale for the nose spray; the patient experiences no allergy response; the patient's skin remains intact; and the patient experiences minimal discomfort.

IMPLEMENTATION

ACTION	RATIONALE
1. Gather equipment. Check medication order against the original order in the medical record, according to facility policy. Clarify any inconsistencies. Check the patient's chart for allergies.	This comparison helps to identify errors that may have occurred when orders were transcribed. The primary care provider's order is the legal record of medication orders for each facility.
2. Know the actions, special nursing considerations, safe dose ranges, purpose of administration, and adverse effects of the medication to be administered. Consider the appropriateness of the medication for this patient.	This knowledge aids the nurse in evaluating the therapeutic effect of the medication in relation to the patient's disorder and can also be used to educate the patient about the medication.
3. Perform hand hygiene.	Hand hygiene prevents the spread of microorganisms.
4. Move the medication cart to the outside of the patient's room or prepare for administration in the medication area.	Organization facilitates error-free administration and saves time.
5. Unlock the medication cart or drawer. Enter pass code and scan employee identification, if required.	Locking the cart or drawer safeguards each patient's medication supply. Hospital accrediting organizations require medication carts to be locked when not in use. Entering pass code and scanning ID allows only authorized users into the system and identifies the user for documentation by the computer.
6. **Prepare medications for one patient at a time.**	This prevents errors in medication administration.
7. Read the CMAR/MAR and select the proper medication from the patient's medication drawer or unit stock.	This is the *first* check of the label.
8. Compare the label with the CMAR/MAR. Check expiration dates and perform calculations, if necessary. Scan the bar code on the package, if required.	This is the *second* check of the label. Verify calculations with another nurse to ensure safety, if necessary.

ACTION

9. Depending on facility policy, the third check of the label may occur at this point. If so, when all medications for one patient have been prepared, recheck the labels with the CMAR/MAR before taking the medications to the patient.

10. Lock the medication cart before leaving it.

11. Transport medications to the patient's bedside carefully, and keep the medications in sight at all times.

12. Ensure that the patient receives the medications at the correct time.

13. Perform hand hygiene and put on PPE, if indicated.

14. Identify the patient. Compare the information with the CMAR/MAR. The patient should be identified using at least two methods (The Joint Commission, 2013):

a. Check the name on the patient's identification band.

b. Check the identification number on the patient's identification band.

c. Check the birth date on the patient's identification band.

d. Ask the patient to state his or her name and birth date, based on facility policy.

15. Complete necessary assessments before administering medications. Check the patient's allergy bracelet or ask the patient about allergies. Explain the purpose and action of each medication to the patient.

16. Scan the patient's bar code on the identification band, if required (Figure 1).

RATIONALE

This *third* check ensures accuracy and helps to prevent errors. *Note:* Many facilities require the *third* check to occur at the bedside, after identifying the patient and before administration.

Locking the cart or drawer safeguards the patient's medication supply. Hospital accrediting organizations require medication carts to be locked when not in use.

Careful handling and close observation prevent accidental or deliberate disarrangement of medications.

Check agency policy, which may allow for administration within a period of 30 minutes before or 30 minutes after the designated time.

Hand hygiene and PPE prevent the spread of microorganisms. PPE is required based on transmission precautions.

Identifying the patient ensures the right patient receives the medications and helps prevent errors. The patient's room number or physical location is not used as an identifier (The Joint Commission, 2013). Replace the identification band if it is missing or inaccurate in any way.

This requires a response from the patient, but illness and strange surroundings often cause patients to be confused.

Assessment is a prerequisite to administration of medications.

Provides an additional check to ensure that the medication is given to the right patient.

FIGURE 1 Scanning bar code on the patient's identification bracelet.

(continued)

SKILL 17 | ADMINISTERING A NASAL SPRAY continued

ACTION

17. Based on facility policy, the third check of the label may occur at this point. If so, recheck the labels with the CMAR/MAR before administering the medications to the patient.

18. Put on gloves.

19. Provide patient with paper tissues and ask the patient to blow his or her nose.

20. Have the patient sit up with head tilted back. **Tilting the patient's head should be avoided if the patient has a cervical spine injury.**

21. Instruct the patient to inhale gently through the nose as the spray is being administered or not to inhale gently as the spray is being administered. Your instruction to the patient will depend on the medication being administered. Consult the manufacturer's instructions for each medication.

22. Agitate the bottle gently, if required for specific medication. Insert the tip of the nosepiece of the bottle into one nostril (Figure 2). Close the opposite nostril with a finger. Instruct the patient to breathe in gently through the nostril, if required. Compress or activate the bottle to release one spray at the same time the patient breathes in.

RATIONALE

Many facilities require the *third* check to occur at the bedside, after identifying the patient and before administration. If facility policy directs the *third* check at this time, this *third* check ensures accuracy and helps to prevent errors.

Gloves protect the nurse from potential contact with contaminants and body fluids.

Blowing the nose clears the nasal mucosa prior to medication administration.

Allows the spray to flow into the nares. Tilting the head is contraindicated with cervical spine injury.

Inhalation helps to distribute the spray in the nares. Inhalation during administration is not recommended for some medications.

Mixes medication thoroughly to ensure a consistent dose of medication.

FIGURE 2 Inserting tip of bottle into one nostril. (From Craven & Hirnle, (2013). *Fundamentals of nursing* (7th ed). Philadelphia: Wolters Kluwer Health/Lippincott Williams & Wilkins, p. 425, Figure 19-8.)

23. Keep the medication container compressed and remove it from the nostril. Release the container from the compressed state. Do not allow the container to return to its original position until it is removed from the patient's nose.

24. Have the patient hold his or her breath for a few seconds, and then breathe out slowly through the mouth. Repeat in the other nostril, as prescribed or indicated.

25. Wipe the outside of the bottle nose piece with a clean, dry tissue or cloth and replace the cap. Instruct the patient to avoid blowing his or her nose for 5 to 10 minutes, depending on the medication.

26. Remove gloves. Assist the patient to a comfortable position.

 27. Remove additional PPE, if used. Perform hand hygiene.

Prevents contamination of the contents of the container.

Allows medication to remain in contact with mucous membranes of nose.

Keeps the end of the bottle clean. Keeps the medication in contact with the mucous membranes of the nose.

This ensures patient comfort.

Removing PPE properly reduces the risk for infection transmission and contamination of other items. Hand hygiene prevents the spread of microorganisms.

ACTION	RATIONALE
28. Document the administration of the medication immediately after administration. See Documentation section below.	Timely documentation helps to ensure patient safety.
29. Evaluate the patient's response to the procedure and medication within an appropriate time frame.	The patient needs to be evaluated for therapeutic and adverse effects from the medication.

EVALUATION

The expected outcomes are met when the patient receives the nose spray successfully; the patient understands the rationale for nose spray; the patient experiences no allergy response; the patient's skin remains intact; and the patient experiences minimal discomfort.

DOCUMENTATION
Guidelines

Document the administration of the medication, including date, time, dose, route of administration, and site of administration, specifically right, left, or both nares, on the CMAR/MAR or record using the required format. If using a bar-code system, medication administration is automatically recorded when the bar code is scanned. PRN medications require documentation of the reason for administration. Prompt recording avoids the possibility of accidentally repeating the administration of the drug. Document pre- and post-administration assessments, characteristics of any drainage, and the patient's response to the treatment, if appropriate. If the drug was refused or omitted, record this in the appropriate area on the medication record and notify the primary care provider. This verifies the reason medication was omitted and ensures that the primary care provider is aware of the patient's condition.

UNEXPECTED SITUATIONS AND ASSOCIATED INTERVENTIONS

- *Patient sneezes immediately after receiving nose spray:* Do not repeat the dosage, because you cannot determine how much medication was actually absorbed.

SPECIAL CONSIDERATIONS

- Ongoing assessment is an important part of nursing care to evaluate patient response to administered medications and early detection of adverse effects. If an adverse effect is suspected, withhold further medication doses and notify the patient's primary care provider. Additional intervention is based on type of reaction and patient assessment.

SKILL VARIATION   Administering Medication via Nasal Drops

Prepare medication as outlined in steps 1–12 above (Skill 17).

1. Perform hand hygiene and put on PPE, if indicated.

2. Identify the patient. The patient should be identified using two methods.

3. Close the door to the room or pull the bedside curtain.
4. **Complete necessary assessments before administering medications. Check allergy bracelet or ask patient about allergies. Explain the purpose and action of the medication to the patient.**
5. Scan the patient's bar code on the identification band, if required.
6. **Based on facility policy, the third check of the label may occur at this point. If so, recheck the labels with the CMAR/MAR before administering the medications to the patient.**

7. Put on gloves. Assist the patient to an upright position with the head tilted back.
8. Draw sufficient solution into the dropper for both nares. Do not return excess solution to the bottle to avoid contamination.
9. Have the patient breathe through the mouth. Hold tip of nose up and place dropper just above naris, about 1/3 inch. Instill the prescribed number of drops in one naris and then into the other. Avoid touching naris with dropper.
10. Have patient remain in position with head tilted back for a few minutes to prevent the escape of the medication.
11. Remove gloves. Assist the patient to a comfortable position.
12. Remove additional PPE, if used. Perform hand hygiene.
13. Document administration of the medication on the CMAR/MAR immediately after administering the medication. Document the site, if only one nostril is used.
14. Evaluate the patient's response to the medication within an appropriate time frame.